Joy in Alzheimer's

My Mom's Brave Walk into Dementia's Abyss

ISBN: 979-8-9987695-1-1 (paperback); 979-8-9987695-0-4 (e-book)

Library of Congress Catalog Number

Cover art in collaboration with Ashely Barron (www.ashleybarronphotography.com)

Editing and Organization in collaboration with Colleen Sell (via Reedsy.com)

First Printing: 2025

29 28 27 26 25 5 4 3 2 1

William C. Barron

Bend, Oregon

simplebender.com

Table of Contents

Joy in Alzheimer's

My Mom's Brave Walk into Dementia's Abyss

William C. Barron

Acknowledgments

Thank you to Jan, my wife, who stood beside Joy and me with patience, understanding, and an empathetic ear and heart. A special thanks as well to our sons and their families, whose many visits, calls, and unwavering support meant more than words can express. This journey would have been a tragedy without them. I am also deeply grateful to all the caregivers at Touchmark Bend who held Joy's hand with compassion throughout her journey.

Have Courage, Be Bold, and **Never Fear the Dream**.

Contents

Prologue

Let's just be honest: there is no joy in Alzheimer's. However, my mom, Joy, was in the middle of it when I became her primary care partner, along with my wife, Jan. So "Joy in Alzheimer's" is where we were and remained for the duration. This book is an attempt to follow her through this unwinnable battle. To open up about how the mental disease affects Joy and those who love and care for her.

Joy was born and raised in far West Texas and lived almost all her life in the greater El Paso valley. She lived in the home she and her husband (my father) designed and built for nearly fifty years. Dad was a stoic realist. He faced death many times as a paratrooper in the 101st, making two of the epic jumps in World War II. He taught his two sons to face obstacles and to be responsible, accountable, and have realistic expectations. He fought cancer for many years, with Joy as his constant, faithful caregiver and support. When he passed, there was an obvious emptiness in Joy's life. But like Dad, she moved on, mourning in her own special way and living alone in the house they built.

In the ensuing years, we began to notice Joy beginning to slip mentally. Physically, she stayed relatively strong and walked almost every day, or so she told us. However, she started to have trouble with directions, driving, remembering details, and following dynamic dialogs. My nephew and his family were stationed in El Paso and lived nearby for several years. To their credit, they reported subtle changes in her mental abilities. Being remote, the rest of the family dismissed the observations. Jan and I rationalized these issues as normal aging ailments; after all, Joy was semi-spry and feisty for her advanced age.

In 2016, ten years after my dad passed and I'd retired, we moved from Alaska to Oregon. Now that Jan and I were back in the continental United States (lower 48) and living in a climate more hospitable for my elderly mom, we invited Joy to leave her longtime home and live in Bend, closer to family. She took her time thinking about the offer and finally accepted with one caveat: "I'm never going to live with you in your home." In early 2017, we sorted out clothes and keepsakes Joy felt she couldn't live without. We loaded her and her treasures into a haul truck and drove across the country. Little did we know it would be one of Joy's last road trips. But it wouldn't be her last journey. Her last journey would be the hardest: her walk into dementia's abyss.

Joy's road, like most with Alzheimer's, started long before anyone really knew. Now that she was living closer to us, we could see some subtle changes that age alone couldn't explain. While Joy was initially the social butterfly in her new residence, sustaining three falls with a head injury just compounded her Alzheimer's problem. She began to lose the ability to pay bills, and her "bookkeeping" went from taking a few hours to taking a few weeks. She started to forget the questions she had just asked, let alone the answers. She began to claim she had spoken with her parents, even though they had long passed.

After a long weekend at her grandson's wedding, thirty minutes into the plane ride home she turned to me: 'Isn't the choir music beautiful?,' she asked. Looking at her, more than a little confused I replied: 'Um sure, do you like it? 'Oh yes, it is wonderful, just wonderful.' she replied. I replied, 'Well good then, just close your eyes and enjoy the choir as long as you want.' The drone of the jet was the only sound anyone could hear, except for Joy. She closed her eyes. A smile came across her lips, and I took a deep breath trying to calm myself. Although her Alzheimer's journey had started many years before, our journey with Joy in Alzheimer's was beginning. While the flight was smooth, I knew our journey was about to get very bumpy. Jan and I were concerned, and even Joy expressed frustration and even anger with her increasing disabilities. Although her journey had started many years before, our journey with Joy in Alzheimer's was just beginning.

PART ONE

Signs of the Journey

Before you start the journey, as best you can, prepare yourself mentally and emotionally for the hardships and unknown.

1

There's No Turning Back Now

Joy transitioned to her new apartment in the independent living facility in Bend with few issues. At the outset, we had many meals with her in the dining room, helping her adjust to a new situation and living conditions. After a week or so, she seemed quite comfortable and flittered around the dining room at each meal like a social butterfly. She was giddy that she didn't have to buy groceries, cook, or clean anymore. She was more outgoing than she had been in years.

But we noticed some changes too. Joy was beginning to misplace things and forgetting to pay bills. She occasionally asked us questions about where her parents and husband were. She would comment that she thought she saw them in the lobby, then giggle and say that was ridiculous and change the subject. We noticed her attention span was decreasing, and she was very easily distracted. She began to shuffle her feet more on her daily walk around the local park. The combination of distractions and shuffling resulted in two hard falls. After some questioning, we learned she had also slipped in the tub a few times.

Joy's life was changing ... and then came COVID. The multi-year isolation was devastating to her social life and confidence. We called her every afternoon at the same time to help build a pattern; even that didn't help. She was losing the concept of time and had lost her ability to manage her finances.

Her third fall, this one on ice and hitting the back of her head, prompted us to take Mom to a neurologist under the pretext of getting a baseline assessment. The appointment went well. The neurologist wasn't overly concerned with her cognitive test results. The diagnosis changed at the next appointment six months later. The doctor was concerned with the delusional episodes and the money-management deterioration, but the illustration below tipped the scales.

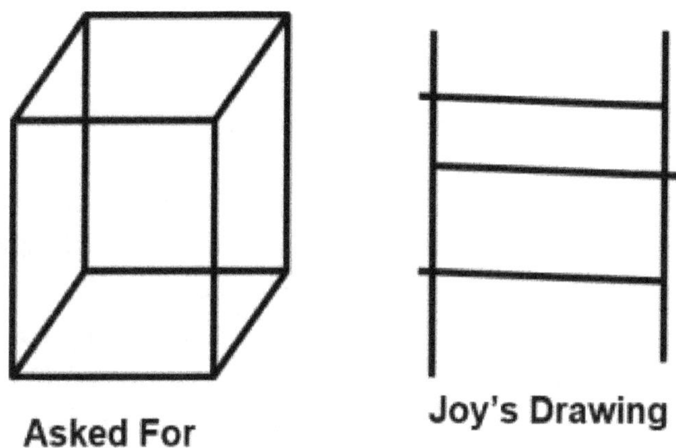

We knew the independent living facility kept a close watch on residents. Following the neurological assessment, we mentioned the diagnoses to them, and they gave us that all-knowing nod. We knew we had to get ahead of the situation. Within six months of that neurological test, we moved Joy to an assisted living facility, before the independent one was forced to ask us to move her. That's where she lived—for more than a year and a half, since the spring of 2022—even though she'd tell you she just moved in, has changed apartments five or six times, and the entire complex has been rotated around several times.

So began our journey with Joy down that long, narrowing path of Alzheimer's. ... A path that no longer had a safety net. ... Where every stumble on her old, uncertain legs and her weakened mind could lead Joy into the deep, dark recesses of dementia.

2

News Is Reality

Today's broadcast news can be best described as depressingly abysmal. For those with Alzheimer's, the pain and confusion caused by watching the televised news can be devastating. This is the case with Joy.

Joy has always been a self-professed "news junkie" and "archivist," someone who always tried to keep up with current events. As a little girl, she sat in front of the radio listening to the reports from Europe about WWII. As an adult, she dutifully watched the evening news with Walter Cronkite and the local news. The Democrat and Republican National Conventions always transfixed her.

But, today, at an increasing frequency, the news she sees has become part of her reality. A terrifying reality. Over the last several years, she mourns for the immigrants, especially those crossing at El Paso, her hometown. We "discuss," to some degree, the state of dysfunction in Washington, D.C., and her disappointment. About a year ago, she started not only empathizing but also internalizing the news and living within it. Her ability to consistently recognize the difference between the news on TV and her life has been sliding down a steep, slippery slope.

The news of college campus shootings resulted in numerous calls to us announcing she was packed and ready to evacuate the "campus" (which is what she calls the assisted living center). The Walmart shooting in El Paso was horrific for her, a delusional trauma that lasted several days before she realized she was not there. She called several times and reported she was just a car away from the President as his motorcade left the DC courthouse for the airport. Why? Because the news was a live broadcast from a car following the motorcade. To her, she was there, in the car, in the motorcade. The wars in Ukraine and Gaza have prompted repeated calls and declarations about wanting to leave and "get away from the big guns and killing down the street." It took almost a week for her to understand the war in Gaza wasn't Jews fighting Jews.

Whatever the tragic, gut-wrenching graphic story of the day might be, she is increasingly likely to believe she is there. She is in the world shown on her TV screen. Joy is most confused and delusional if she is dozing in her recliner with the news blaring into her subconscious. When her slumber ends, Joy is in the world she's been hearing and now seeing.

All efforts by her doctors, facility care team, and us to turn off the TV have been summarily rejected. As she says, "I'm running the world, and it's in a mell of a hess." I understand, I really do. Watching TV is about all she's got left to do. She remembers little of what she reads, so she doesn't make the effort. The assisted living facility has a bounty of activities accommodating people with light memory loss. Unfortunately, she chooses not to take part. Self-isolation and the horrendously graphic news are not a good combination. I don't like what it is doing to what's left of her mind and her emotions. At this point, the delusions last a day or so, but the duration is slowly increasing.

We have decided not to try and jar her from that reality. Instead, we try to try and soothe her nerves and anxiety, using calm words and distracting her with other more pleasant subjects. Sometimes it works; sometimes it doesn't.

3

Just Answer, Don't Argue

Robust discussions were commonplace in my parents' home. Joy always enjoyed a good, non-emotional, intellectual discussion. She was adept at formulating words to thrust and parry through a complex subject. She wouldn't hesitate to artfully turn my words against me or suddenly change sides to take me off balance.

That's who she was; that is no longer who she is. I've come to the realization, through several knots on my metaphorical head, that challenging discussions simply upset her. Before each phone call or visit, we remind ourselves, "Just answer the question, and don't argue." It's just not worth the unintended pain I hear and see.

We've learned the hard way not to argue with Joy and not to correct her, unless we absolutely have to for her safety and care. Arguing puts too much emotional strain on all of us. Before we knew Joy had Alzheimer's, our Sunday evening dinners became exceedingly difficult. She would descend into emotional, illogical arguments over issues big and small. Had we known then what we know now, we would have done things differently. We now practice the subtle art of distraction and agreement. Sadly, the hope for delightfully engaging Sunday dinners has disappeared.

Joy has lost the ability to formulate linked cognitive thoughts for any semblance of a dialog. Her world is closing in, and she can only deal with immediate things. We have learned to give her two choices and let her choose. We've learned it's better to quietly nod as she espouses political or philosophical opinions. We have learned to distract and defer rather than confront. She's pleasant enough as her reality becomes confused with the upsetting news she watches.

In response to Joy's tangled monologue concerning "terrorists on campus," intermixed with asking about the family's health, we calmly just try to answer the question. On the fifth inquiry regarding the kids' health in under five minutes, we assure her they are still okay.

Joy calls and exclaims she is dressed, outside, waiting for us, and ready for her doctor's appointment.

"Where are you?" she asks.

This isn't the first time this has happened. Knowing she doesn't have an appointment, we respond, "Isn't it tomorrow? We'll call the doctor to make sure."

Our follow-up call to her a few moments later is either, "The doctor called and apologized, but he had to postpone your appointment," or "Your appointment is tomorrow; is that okay?" She seems quite satisfied, and we move along.

Recently, at dinner, she said, "It's good to be back home."

Knowing she hadn't been anywhere, we asked if she'd had a good time.

She emphatically said. "Yes, a wonderful time," but she couldn't tell us where she'd gone.

We've learned to ask her questions rather than make statements. It's so much easier and less contentious.

She often says her "mama and daddy" are in town, demanding she go home with them and be their "little girl" again. It doesn't matter that they died over thirty years ago. She asks if we've seen them. We tell her we've not seen them in a long time, and she shouldn't worry about going home with them. She is safe and comfortable where she is and needs to be. Exasperated, she is emphatic that "Mama" always gets her way. We give her more reassurance, and then we try to divert her focus on bygone times by asking how her walk or lunch was today. Sometimes it works. Sometimes, it doesn't, and we make another lap around the "mama and daddy" track.

We no longer tell her that her parents and her husband have passed away. We stopped doing that when we started to hear and see the depression we were causing by being too honest about those losses.

Now, if she stumbles upon the realization of their passing, that's okay; if not, that's all right, too.

It is like being a little rubber duck floating down a river, bumping into rocks and jetsam and being pulled into eddies. The rubber duck doesn't care; it's along for the ride, and so are we. We recognize that Joy's mind confuses time and people now, and we just go with the flow.

4

I've Become My Dad

When we are young, time seems to move at glacial speed or to stand still. When we age, time seems to fly by, to pass in the blink of an eye. For Joy and other Alzheimer's patients, time is like watching a tub drain, with time swirling around and around, mixing the past and the present into an undistinguishable blur.

For Joy, places and people are now increasingly a blur, and their interconnection often confuses her. She celebrated her ninetieth birthday this year (2023), and the entire family was able to attend the celebration. Over the few days of activities Joy would pull different people aside and ask, "Who belongs to who?" In all fairness, at ninety, we would all have some trouble remembering the family members who live all over the country, spanning three generations, with very few having had an opportunity to visit. The good news is we had a wonderful reunion; the bad news is the resulting fatigue and confusion for Joy, which lasted for several months. Even now, ten months later, any mention of a birthday or any flowers she receives are "obviously" for her birthday, which "was just the other day." She is so cute and happy to think she has such a frequent special occasion.

Joy now blends stories and concerns about her deceased parents with today's events. She weaves intricate stories of how her deceased brother and parents are contriving to take her back to El Paso. But the breath was taken out of us when she called a few months ago and asked, "Where is your father?" My dad passed away from cancer over fifteen years ago. We were stammering and, unfortunately, said he had passed away. We will never, ever, do that again. The despair and anguish we heard on the phone was heartbreaking. My mom's voice broke and cracked as she asked when he'd died, and upon hearing he'd passed away in 2006, the phone was silent for a long time. She then asked, "Where have I been all this time?"

Almost every week now, we get the question of my father's location, whether he will be home for dinner, or whether she should order him some dinner. Every time, we do a little verbal dance and change the subject.

The most breathtaking moment was the day I became my dad. My mom called unexpectedly, and when I answered, she responded in a very terse, arsenic-laden voice:

Mom "This is your *wife*! Where are you? Are Mama and Daddy with you? Did you have a good time without me?"

Me "Well, of course not."

Mom "Fine, I forgive you."

We then asked how her walk was and how many geese she had seen. Just as fast as I was my dad, I was again her son. We had dodged another bullet.

It isn't that, to my knowledge, my dad did anything for her to question in their 54 years of marriage; it's that she thought she had been left out.

Now, in conversations with Joy, my identity routinely swings between me being her son and me being her husband in the same half hour. I am quizzed about my (his) location and/or if I am (he is) coming home for dinner. One never knows how to respond when you have a forced split personality. There is a genuine concern whether Joy is losing her pleasant personality and becoming increasingly biting, upset, and terse. It happens, and we now must prepare ourselves for such a possibility.

Blending time and people, the living and the dead is now a common occurrence for Joy. The stories swirl between current events and the ever-extending distant past, with the recent past almost forgotten. There does seem to be a reasonable correlation between her confusion and fatigue and the time of day, which is the classic "sundowners" people with Alzheimer's often experience.

5

Delirium

For some time, Joy has had sporadic events of seeing, hearing, and/or feeling things that are not there, but the last two weeks have been especially challenging for her. Last week, she called almost every day, expressing disappointment that we hadn't spoken in several weeks. She insisted she had spoken with "Mama and Daddy" but not to us.

This week, we slid down the slope a little farther and a little faster. We called her midday on Sunday to arrange our typical weekend pizza dinner.

A few hours later, she called and asked, "Where are you? Where did you go? You were just here, and then you suddenly left. Did I upset you?"

We said we were at home watching football. Then it dawned on us: Joy thought we had been in her room and left unexpectedly without telling her. We hadn't been to her room. So, in the spirit of answering and not arguing, we added, "You seemed to doze off, so we slipped out to get ready for our pizza dinner."

The next day came her panicked call, declaring, "Hamas has invaded! They are bombing the city and destroying the hospital! We have to evacuate and escape!"

We took the call while shopping. We must have looked odd, our heads together trying to hear without being on speaker, calmly telling Mom we were all safe, over and over again.

This was followed by the evening call, "Where are you? I was sitting on the couch talking with Mama and Daddy, and you left. Is everything all right?"

We assured her everything was fine.

"I forgive you," she responded.

Then, there was Halloween morning. She called in a panic, terrified, her voice quivering and slurring a little. "They're packing my stuff, and Mama is moving me. They are saying the lockbox won't open. The lady is here with fancy cowboy boots and is packing me and giving me medication."

We spoke some calming words, which seemed to appease her. Then, we sent a quick text message to the nurse's station. They apologetically replied that the medical technician was dressed in Western wear for Halloween, which confused Joy.

We'd no sooner caught our breath before we got another panic call from Joy.

"I don't know what's going on. I don't know what the plan is, but I know Mama is pulling strings to move me."

Our reassuring words slowly calmed her back down. Seemingly, we'd convinced her that her mother would be almost 120 years old, and we didn't think she could be instigating any move.

Bear in mind that these are not five-minute phone calls. They all last 15–30 minutes or more, each and every one of them, as we take countless laps around the figure eight infinity loop. In this case, it turns out, the medical technician had startled her from sleep and was dressed in Rodeo attire for Halloween. The next several calls from Joy were much better, but she was still fixated on my grandmother's conspiracy to move her.

The sad part is that the more she has these delusional episodes, the closer she gets to having to move to memory care. Ironically, a move is in her near future, but one instigated not by her mother but by her condition and actions.

As hard as these episodes are for us, they must be absolutely mind-shattering for Mom. To hear the panic and fear in her voice is breathtaking and heartbreaking. The delusions must be just terrifying to her. For Joy, we and the caretakers at the facility are her lifeline and support, always on hand. For us and other caregivers, we need to find and use resources of our own, to help guide and sustain us.

6

Jamais Vu: Darn Phone

We've discovered a term that describes a lot of what Joy is going through. *Jamais vu* means experiencing a familiar situation as unfamiliar. It is like encountering something you've known forever for the first time. This must be what Joy feels every time she tries to use her phone.

Keep in mind that Joy is approaching 91 years old. She grew up using a phone hung on the wall and being connected by an operator. As technology changed, she did, too. She loved the idea of talking on a long-distance call as soon as they were cheaper than letters. For years and years, she's been able to use a phone. She transitioned to cell phones and then smartphones, and she semi-mastered texting and even surfing the internet on her smartphone.

But now, Jamais Vu has taken hold, and the phone is becoming a mystery and a challenge. It is no longer an extension of her, but rather an unworkable device that demands too much to remember. Portable phones are things of science fiction, while phones on your wrist, well, those are things out of Dick Tracy and the comics. She has two phones: an older model iPhone that uses a home button and a portable phone in the apartment. We've posted critical phone numbers on cards and placards in her apartment. We've ensured her contact list is up-to-date and her "favorites" are easy to find. Every week, and sometimes every day, we are reminded that what seems easy for us is so complicated for her. The simple process of opening the phone and dialing one with a keypad is now a significant chore.

Recently, while Joy was on her cell phone with us, she exasperatedly exclaimed that her cell phone wasn't working anymore ... while she was using it. We suggested she bring it to dinner that evening, and we'd take a look.

We sat down for pizza, Joy's Sunday Favorite. Suddenly, she reached into her purse and pulled out her TV remote.

Mom Shaking the phone in the air. "It just won't work when I punch in the numbers!"

Me Looking at the remote, taking a deep breath: "Umm, that thing doesn't work at all well as a phone, but it works great telling your TV what to do."

Mom Not missing a beat: "I just can't get it to work when I call you."

Me "Yep, you should really use that only for the TV and use your cell phone to call us."

Mom "Well, it's worked before. But that other phone doesn't work at all with the TV!"

Me "Wouldn't think so, but you can call me on the other one and use the one in your hand for the TV. It'll work great."

A few more laps, and it seemed to slowly sink in.

We no longer call her cell phone and only call her portable "house" phone. We are pretty confident we will find her sitting in her recliner watching the news with the portable phone in its cradle next to her. The green answer button is hard to miss. There's no telling where the cell phone might be at any given moment or whether she'll be able to swipe it correctly to answer a call. We know her ability to call out on it is all but gone. As she would say, she "needs a lesson." There's just one problem: with Alzheimer's, once you forget how to do something, it is almost impossible to re-learn it. The memory just doesn't stick around. However, she seems thrilled when, by chance, she can get the cell phone to work, which makes her happy for that moment.

Jamais vu at its finest. Something so familiar yet so foreign all at the same time.

Her frustration at times is just crippling and demoralizing to her. She knows she used to know, and it's crushing. Her self-confidence is shattered, and her frustration and anger rise to the surface. Fortunately, she rarely remembers these frustrating times. She just gets to repeat them over and over again.

We've noticed the adverse effects of fatigue, especially in the evenings. Some specialists call this "sundowners." We call it "Cognitive Exhaustion."

7
Cognitive Exhaustion

Mom is beleaguered with a part of Alzheimer's that is quite common and very disturbing. Widely called *sundowners*, it refers to a period of any given day during which Alzheimer's patients are particularly susceptible to confusion and delirium. Typically, this occurs at the end of the day as the sun is going down.

Because this affects Joy not only in the evenings but also after extra stimulation, we tend to refer to it as *Cognitive Exhaustion*. Can you imagine the energy and focus required to do everything you can every moment of the day to maintain your dignity as you lose your continence, confidence, common sense, and memory? It must be exhausting. Even if you still had a little of your youth and stamina, it would be exhausting. For some, a night's rest is enough to reset and recharge. For Joy, that's not always the case, and some of her episodes of sundowners are particularly devastating and last for days.

Think about yourself and how hard it is to make decisions when you are tired. Coach Lombardi is credited with saying, "Fatigue will make cowards of the strongest." We've all experienced uncertainty and self-doubt when physically or mentally tired. But most of us haven't lost our continence and the self-confidence that results. We haven't lost our ability to calmly assess a situation and employ common sense to resolve issues. Most of us can still lean upon our memories to help make sense of issues and use those recollections to support our opinions and decisions. Alzheimer's patients either have lost or are losing all of those. Now, all their energy is spent just trying to hang on with a modicum of dignity. As the day ends, their minds have reached a level of exhaustion that increases their dementia. Like an endurance athlete at the end of a race, whose muscles are spent and failing along with other bodily and mental functions, so it is with victims of Alzheimer's. Only for them, cognitive exhaustion happens every day, day after day.

We have noticed that multi-day events are particularly disastrous for Joy. We have learned to keep her participation down to a few hours at a time and then return her to her apartment, her quiet space, to rest. Sometimes, she returns to activities; sometimes, she doesn't. It depends on how she feels or how confused she appears. Even with these precautions, a few days of a higher level of activity has an extended impact on Mom. It is as if the stimulus, as enjoyable as it is, has a compounding effect. Imagine how difficult it would be to try as hard as you can to remember names, to "not say something stupid," and to be socially engaged while not having an "accident."

After too much stimulation and the effort Joy expended trying to keep up, naps and evening sleep usually do not rest her mind or emotions. Her cognitive exhaustion is compounding and challenging to overcome. What used to take her a few days to recover is now taking a week or more. Desperate, panicked phone calls are now the norm following these events. Joy enjoys family activities. She wants to be involved and be a part of the party. The good news is she does not seem to understand or remember the consequences. So, in the end, it is all worthwhile.

PART TWO

Memory Playing Tricks

It's best to have a clear, realistic view of delusion, not a delusional perspective of reality.

8
Lost in Plain Sight

One of the interesting aspects of Alzheimer's, beyond memory loss, is the victim's gradual loss of visual recognition—the ability to recognize and identify what is in plain sight. In some cases, their field of vision continually degrades. That is the case with Joy. This degradation, on top of age-related visual deterioration, creates a setting that can be absolutely debilitating. Joy's macular degeneration certainly does not help.

We noticed Joy was having trouble finding things in her apartment. We thought it was because she did not remember where she put them. Then, while we were with her at the grocery store, letting her try to do some shopping, she stood staring at the toothpaste section for an extended time. Trying hard not to interfere, I stood just behind her for what seemed like an eternity. She finally turned and, with an exasperated voice, said she couldn't find her brand. Knowing what she wanted, we were taken aback because her choice was directly in front of her, at eye level—hidden in plain sight. At the time, we thought the magnitude of toothpaste selection was so great that it totally overwhelmed her. But as time has progressed, we are recognizing there is a vision component that must be addressed.

We take Joy to her ophthalmologist and retina specialist on a routine schedule. Technically, her vision has not changed in several years. Her macular degeneration has not progressed much, and her correction prescription has not changed at all for several years. But she simply cannot see or recognize items around her. After some research, I discovered that Alzheimer's indeed affects the field of vision. At least two issues collude to make visual acuity more complex: (1) The patient develops a narrowing of the field of vision. Slowly, the vision pattern becomes more tunnel-like, as if the camera's aperture is closing and peripheral views are being shut out. (2) The patient's mind is having more difficulty making the connection between what is seen and what the objects are. They may see it but not readily recognize it. After a moment or two of focus, Joy can still make the visual-mental connection, for now.

She will frantically search for items in her small apartment and not see they are in plain sight. Getting her on the right calendar is a good example. Finding the calendar is the first hurdle. We then patiently ensure she is on the correct year and then the right month to note something on the right day. She refuses to discard calendars, so finding the correct year is sometimes the biggest hurdle. She will stare at the date and simply not recognize the numbers or the connection with this year's date. Ensuring she is on the correct year, month, and day to note an appointment has taken more than half an hour. We resist doing it for her. She feels so noble once she's accomplished the task. Using that information on the appointed day is an entirely different issue.

Joy maintains a reasonably good sense of humor despite these visual deficiencies. We are now accustomed to hearing, "All the Christmas decorations are in the storage shed. I've turned this apartment upside down a dozen times. They simply are not here." Only to hear a few days later how happy she is that the apartment is fully decorated for the holidays. Now, if only we can get her to understand Christmas isn't tomorrow or yesterday or every other day.

9
Episodic Memory

There is so much to learn along this journey. There is so much you never wanted to learn. There is so much you learn by observation. So much you really must learn, even if you don't want to. We watch Joy slowly slip away and are delighted by the times she is right there with us. We watch her internal clock of memories rewind slowly and then get jumbled with current events. We have decided her episodic memory is simply all messed up. We do not think she has necessarily "lost memory." Joy cannot recall what she wants in the time sequence she needs.

In trying to understand memory, we have discovered some things. We have learned that there are two primary forms of memory: explicit and implicit. *Explicit memory* is the memory of events. These are stored in the hippocampus, neocortex, and amygdala, which are the primary target of Alzheimer's. *Implicit memory*, the target of Parkinson's, is the memory of motor skills and is stored in the cerebellum and basal ganglia.

Explicit memory is subdivided into episodic and semantic memory. *Episodic memory* is formed by the events you experience and lessons you have learned, which are linked in a chronological time reference. These memories are created and stored in the hippocampus, backed-up during sleep to the neocortex, and also stored in the amygdala, which attaches emotional significance to the memories. *Semantic memory* is a recall of knowledge of facts, not necessarily time-related.

The linking of memory with time is so critical as Alzheimer's progresses. It is unclear if the memories are actually erased or if they aren't readily accessed as plaque builds up on the receptors. In Joy's case, it seems as if the memories are there, but their chronological order and emotional relevance are scrambled. Joy's primary timeframe of discussion is her childhood and her relationship with her parents, although viewed almost in the third person with analysis. She will be telling 75-year-old stories about her "mama and daddy" and then intermix a few about a friend from last year or her discussion with the caregivers this morning. She ties them all together as if they were integral to each other and the overall story.

Joy will often ask for cell phone or laptop "lessons." After repeated tutorials going over the same material, we have recognized that her ability to form short-term memories and to routinely recall them is essentially gone. This fits with a common observation of Alzheimer's patients that we describe as "you cannot relearn a skill you've lost"—no matter the volume of copious notes Joy takes. First, she must find the notes, and by then she is too tired to try or forgets why she was looking for them. She "punches" around on the phone until she manages to make a call. But the laptop is a hopeless case and is relegated to a back corner in her apartment.

Joy is trying so hard. We watch her clench her fist in frustration as she tries to recall family names or situations. She remains very pleasant to the caregivers, but we can tell the aggravation and deep-seated emotional scars are being exposed with every passing story. But then, the next day, she usually does not recall any agitation and peacefully asks who is visiting our house. She always seems surprised no one is here for the Holidays because she often thinks Christmas is tomorrow, or yesterday, or last week.

10

Twelve Days of Christmas

The holiday season has brought Joy little peace, calm, or joy this year. The twelve days of Christmas have been fraught with uncertainty, confusion, and despair, with only a few respites of calm and assurance. Over the last few years, we have noticed the holiday season is becoming harder and harder for Joy. Holiday activities in the halls disrupt her normal routines—her self-imposed duty to decorate her apartment and think about holiday cards and gifts, only to be disappointed in her inability to accomplish anything and confusion with so many things.

Joy is not alone in feeling stress and disorientation during the holiday season. Even people without Alzheimer's or mental illness are pushed to the brink with the expectations and traditions of this time of year. It is as if we have forgotten the reason for the season. And when Joy watches the news, she certainly does not see any peace, joy, or thanksgiving in the world she immerses herself in. In this regard, some of Joy's confusion is not her fault. Good grief, the TV ads for Christmas shopping started before Halloween! No wonder she starts out confused, like a lot of us.

For Joy, her emotions are caught up in the blender of her memory. Over the last two weeks, she has had a recurring fear of her "mama" orchestrating and manipulating her life and her accommodations. In call after call, she says she is boxing up her Christmas decorations and starting to pack because "Mama is moving me back to Texas, but I don't want to go." Repeated reassurance, the facade of calm, appears to help ... until she stumbles into the realization her parents are dead. This epiphany yields a sigh of relief. However, the sigh is quickly followed by, "I know where they are buried, and we had a nice chat yesterday."

The twelve days of Christmas have been a series of packing and unpacking, putting up and taking down decorations, boxing pictures, and then putting them back on the nightstand. This routine has been eclipsed only by the complete disorientation of time. She does not understand why no one is in town for the holidays. After all, Christmas was last week, or it's tomorrow, or it was yesterday. And she keeps telling the caregivers, "Happy New Year! I'll be moving soon."

She has called numerous times asking, "Where are you?" as she sits in the cold vestibule for the ride, which was never discussed or planned. The sad truth is she will be moving soon, not to Texas, but to memory care. At times, she is cognitive enough to understand where her degradation is taking her, and she expresses anger at her loss and at her future.

Joy used to love Christmas. Singing in the choir, making cookies, candies, and fruit cakes, decorating the house, and eagerly waiting for family to arrive. But now the holiday seems like more of a duty than a pleasure, a duty even though she does not know when it is or where she will be. We will do what we can to make the time special as well as restful, but those might be mutually exclusive competing goals. The time following the Holidays will be the most trying, as Joy fights fatigue and bewilderment and awakens to a new world after each nap.

11
Post-Nap Delusions

Awakening from a nice nap or restful night's slumber clears our heads and refreshes our tired bodies. For Joy, that is not necessarily the case, and it seems the deeper her fatigue, the more vivid her dreams and the more salient her delusions upon waking. Your mind needs to rest and sort out events and emotions. Unfortunately for Joy, those dreams are very real until she has at least one cup of coffee.

We have fielded phone calls that start with, "Where did you go? You were just here. How did you slip out? I just laid down for a quick rest." Or, "Mama and Daddy and my brother (with a sneer in her voice) were here just a moment ago; are they with you?" After a bit of light questioning, we discover she has just risen from a nap. Typically, her rest was interrupted and restless, and she is sitting in her recliner still drowsy and in the brain fog of semi-slumber. It's taken some time, but we've learned not to snap her back to reality quickly but to meet her halfway and slowly bring her around. Sometimes it works; sometimes it does not. Either way, it is all right, as long as she is comfortable and her mind and emotions are calm.

Now that we are on the outer edge of post-Christmas decompression, we are watching her mind push further back in time while stirring in a healthy dose of the present. She seemed to enjoy the festivities with family, but you could see her slowly losing energy and clarity. Even with a three-hour nap before dinner, her time and location disorientation were very apparent when she awakes. To her credit and the family's patience, she powered through and genuinely seemed to savor the family time.

However, the days since have been hard for her and are giving us an indication of the struggles we all have ahead of us. Picking her up for dinner, she looked at us with a distant look of *I know you, I think, but why are you here?* So we began the slow dance into the middle ground of reality, allowing her the chance to gain some confidence and composure before seeing others. Fortunately, the themes are similar; they are just more profound. Since Christmas she has been trying to call my father, worried he might not be all right, expressing resentment he isn't sleeping in her bed. On the telephone, she confuses me with him, referring to me as her "boyfriend" and "love." It is touching that she still thinks of him with such passion. We simply tell her he is all right and in a much better place. The times she remembers his death are becoming increasingly infrequent.

The sad part is that since Christmas, she has routinely expressed great disappointment that she spent Christmas alone while the family celebrated, or she asks why no one has called or is going to pick her up for the party. We have tried to explain that she did have Christmas with the family. We show her pictures and videos, see her face lighten up and then fade. Then we let it go and try to console her. And we relish the moments of clarity.

PART THREE

Learning to Accept

Learn to accept yourself as you learn to accept others, especially those you love.

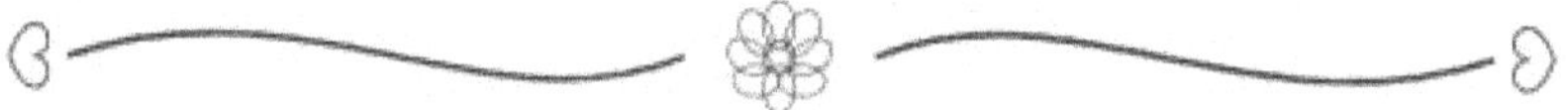

12

Moments of Clarity

As time passes, Joy's moments of clarity are becoming fewer. But when they are there, they are celebrated, even if it is heartbreaking. This is one of the most confusing aspects of Alzheimer's, at least for us. At times, it is just so hard to know if the story Mom is telling is totally real or partially. So far, we do not believe we have witnessed complete fabrication. A shifting mosaic of past, present, and hallucinations is usually the hand we are dealt. We try to play it the best we can, allowing her to believe we believe.

Joy deserves a lot of credit. She does have a fantastic five-minute story to tell. Outwardly, it is always upbeat and positive. She is so good at this five-minute spiel that new staff members are convinced she doesn't need to be in light memory care. She genuinely tries to live up to her name and bring joy to those she encounters. But privately, to us, her moments of clarity are much darker, more confused, and show her loss of confidence, value, and dignity. She shares with us her fears and her confusion. wrapped together and held in place by smaller and smaller strips of reality.

"I'm slipping and can no longer do even the simple things I used to be able to do." That recent moment of clarity was almost haunting in its accuracy.

Alzheimer's clouds Joy's memory so much now. She becomes agitated and distraught with things that exist only in her imagination, but are really her reality. The anxiety of her mother's domination and control. The anger, long buried deep in her core, of her perception of inequitable treatment between her and her brother. She occasionally acknowledges the death of her parents, brother, and husband and yet is absolutely convinced she talked with them "just the other day," either in person or on the phone. It is not about her not accepting their death and moving on. It is about their memories cycling through her mind and recurring at the oddest times.

As many times as Joy fondly mentions my father, she also comes out with, "He didn't love me how I wanted to be loved." She promptly changes the subject and moves on, as if her pronouncement would be accepted as fact. So now we metaphorically scratch our heads, wondering whether she was having a moment of clarity or disorientation. We may never know. Honestly, we really do not want to know. Maybe our reality doesn't need to be distorted by hers, or perhaps it does.

13
Paranoia

Joy's moments of clarity are clouded more than ever by the ever-thickening veil of confusion. Yet, the confusion is leading down a darker path of paranoia, and she is beginning to act as if her nightmares are real.

Paranoia is an unrealistic fear or concern that harm is imminent or others are out to get you. Unfortunately, it is a common trait associated with late-middle and late-stage Alzheimer's. While unrealistic to us, the fear and anxiety a person with Alzheimer's suffers is very real. Like many characteristics of Alzheimer's, some suffer from paranoia, and some do not. As their memory fades, the bonds of emotions remain. The whisperings of the past creep into the forefront of their being, and age-old feelings, festerings, and anxieties begin to emerge. At first, your light touch and soft calming words can help drive away their imagined ghosts. As the paranoia deepens, acting on those whisperings becomes a real problem. So now it is with Joy.

As you may have gathered, Joy's "mama and daddy" make frequent appearances in her altered reality—whisperings from the past brought forward sometimes with pleasure but mostly with anxiousness. Joy adored her father and had some uncomfortable encounters with her mother, who she feels was a controlling and manipulating person. Joy has had recurring awakening dreams about her mother coming to the care center and demanding she leave with her to take care of her parents.

These dreams have become very real to Joy in the last few weeks. Real to the extent she is now taking physical action in response to this paranoia. She has begun to literally pack suitcases for her impending trip. She has removed pictures from her walls and bookcases and stored them in boxes. Joy has announced to the care team, as she packs, that she is "leaving with Mama because she's demanding I go." Her room is becoming disheveled as various articles of clothing end up in odd places, and some are never seen again. Joy calls us, on the verge of tears, shaking with emotion, begging us, "Don't let Mama take me. I just don't want to go." We continually tell her she is not leaving and that we will take care of everything. We help her unpack and set things back in their place as best we can (and still wonder where she put all her underwear). We hope she doesn't take these actions any further, like walking out with a packed suitcase. It has been minus 7 degrees here for the last few days, and she doesn't have an appreciation of temperature anymore, a physical sensation that has long been lost.

As Joy's ability to, as she says, "sober up" from the state of paranoia and dementia also begins to fail her, we have started to wonder: Is she really afraid? Or is she, in her own way, trying to make sure her parents are cared for as she emotionally and mentally prepares for her own departure? Is she trying to sort through the confusion and making her own final arrangements? Or is she just terrified, and her living terror keeps getting stronger and longer and more salient?

Paranoia is a terrible symptom of Alzheimer's and dementia. The person experiencing paranoia *believes* the imagined threats they "hear" and "see" and "feel" are actually happening. That triggers their fear, anger, worry, or other emotional distress. And they respond accordingly. Paranoia steals their sense of well-being and changes their behavior. Just terrible.

Hand in hand, the journey continues.

14

It's Not What You Say, But How You Say It

Over the last few years, one thing has become more evident: It is not what Jan and I say but how we say it that matters when speaking with Joy. For all practical purposes, my mom has lost most of her ability to separate the events of the past from those of the present. She often takes simple clarifying questions as challenges and retorts, "You expect me to remember? You know my memory is shot!"

What we found to be more effective is pretty simple but complicated to execute: speaking in calm tones—nothing harsh, quick, or brisk, just soft, slow, and soothing.

Before Jan and I call or visit my mom, we remind and reinforce ourselves so that one of us can be face-to-face with Joy and speak with gentle, placating tones. Our goal is not to question, challenge, or say something that might make her feel she has to defend herself. We could tell her almost anything in those tones, and between her hearing loss and dementia, there is little fear of a negative reaction. It does happen, and then we calmly apologize for any misunderstanding we might have caused. Then, we smile and try to change the subject to anything else. It does not matter who initiated the tension. It is easier and more expedient to apologize and then move on. Within a few moments, Joy does not recall what the kerfuffle was about or that there was one, and it all seems right in her world. And that is what is important.

Then, when you least expect it, you realize the impact of words.

Joy called, distraught, searching for my dad. She said she'd been with him at noon, and he'd gone down to the lobby, and she'd told the staff he was missing. She expressed concern about getting him a meal and bringing it back to the room. We assured her Dad was fine and suggested she get one meal, and when he shows up, get another. An hour or so later, she called again:

Mom "Where is your father? I'm serious!"

We were concerned she would go looking for him, and it was below zero outside.

Me Reluctantly and in the most calm, soft tone I could muster: "Mom, Dad is in a better place."

Mom Deafening silence, then a gasp, a choke, and a shaking voice: "I was with him at noon. Oh wait, I remember, he died a few months ago. Yes, I remember now. I guess I'll go get one meal."

Thirty minutes later, Joy calls again.

Mom "He was a good man and a good father, but he passed about six months ago, right?"

Me "Mom, Dad passed over fifteen years ago."

Mom Another gasp, silence, then choking words: "Oh, I remember, taking him back to El Paso and the staff being so nice."

Me "Yes, Mom, you were at the service, and it was nice."

It was all right for Mom to remember it that way; it made her feel better. There was no need to remind her that Dad passed away in El Paso many years before she moved to Oregon.

Sometimes words do matter, but we could not let her hurt herself in her quest to find him. Sometimes, in the moment, you just cannot find the right words, and sometimes those words bring pain. In general, though, calm, kind words get us through most of the speedbumps, and most of Joy's days pass uneventfully.

15

Seeking Relevancy

We want to make a few things clear. People with Alzheimer's or dementia are suffering from cognitive decline.

They are not stupid.

They can still think.

They still have deep emotions.

They can still sense your feelings.

They, too, want to be relevant in their world.

Just because it takes them longer to process information and formulate a response does not mean they cannot. As Alzheimer's and dementia deepen, they may eventually just give up trying because of the strain, frustration, and perceived failure. Just because their episodic memory returns information with the consistency of a random number generator or a light through a kaleidoscope does not mean they are not trying.

Like all of us, they want and need a sense of relevancy in their lives. These people were successful in their profession, in raising families, in their communities, and in surviving some of the most turbulent times in history. They still want to have a purpose in life. However small that purpose might seem to us, it is huge for them. If you think small things are irrelevant, you obviously haven't spent much time contemplating a mosquito.

So it is with Joy. She adamantly and repeatedly proclaims, "I don't want to be a burden." Being a burden to her means losing all sense of independence and self-value. For most of Joy's life, she has been the one to give comfort and support—either to her family or friends in need. She gave without asking for anything in return, except maybe a simple thank you. Now, she is on the receiving end of the care and support, and she struggles with the feeling of dependency. It agitates her at times and depresses her at others.

Joy's new life's mission is to bring cookies to non-ambulatory people who seem lonely and/or depressed. This is her way of being relevant and bringing joy. She started being the "Cookie Monster," as she declared after she tried to brighten the day of a bedridden resident by bringing her cookies. That pleased Joy so much that she started working with the facility kitchen and care team, and she now delivers cookies to folks in both the Assisted Living and Memory Care units. This is her niche in her community, and she is thrilled when people "light up light big sunflowers" when she gives them a cookie.

It is a simple act of giving and receiving, of being kind to one another when both the giver and receiver are down. There is a huge lesson here for all of us. In Joy's simple task of delivering a simple cookie, she shows we are all part of humanity every day, and a little kindness can pierce some extremely hard armor.

When Joy's ailing friend passed away, Joy took it hard. She lost her first cookie customer and friend at the facility. Since then, she has felt tired, and as of yet, she is unmotivated to renew her Cookie Monster role. We encourage her with soft supportive words, and we see the glimmer of her need for relevancy bubbling back to the surface. It will take time, but Joy will rebound to some degree.

16
Sliding Backward

The New Year has not been kind to Joy. There was so much excitement and fatigue generated by the holidays. There were the calls and well wishes for her ninety-first birthday. Then, there was the loss of her first friend and Cookie Monster customer. All of these have played a part in where Joy's mind is today.

We have become increasingly concerned with my mom's situation. For the past three to four weeks, she has called us every afternoon, asking, "Where the family is," and "What are the plans for dinner?" For a while, we thought she was referring to our immediate family. She had seen them at Christmas; we thought this was a lingering memory. We were wrong.

After some careful questioning, we discovered she was referring to her parents. Every afternoon, we explained they were not here and that we had not seen or talked with them for several years. We've repeatedly made overt and direct comments about them not being around, but we never said they were deceased. A few months ago, Joy would have finally "heard" us and understood the situation, but no longer.

We arranged a meeting with her care team leader and expressed our concern. She said the team was concerned as well. We discussed the precursors and timing of moving Joy from assisted living to memory care. The message was simple. They look at two things with Joy:

1. Whether she still knows the difference between assisted living and memory care
2. Whether she has demonstrated she's a risk to herself or others

We struggle a little with the first criteria. If she were to move, she could see herself as someone who could help others and embrace it.

Conversely, she could see herself as someone who doesn't belong and become bitter. We believe the latter concerns the facility.

At this week's Sunday dinner, Joy was adamant that my cousin, father, and her parents had been in her room most of the day. She was so convinced that she got up from the table and headed back to her room to bring them to dinner.

She returned a little confused. "I do not know where they went, but they are in the building somewhere. We should order them dinner."

We suggested we order when they arrive.

As the dinner finished, she said, "The only thing that would have made this better is if your brother and father had been here and not walked off."

We agreed and hugged her. She mumbled something about needing to go look for them and her parents. We motioned to a staff caregiver to ensure she made it back to her room.

Once again, her "normal" has changed, and we must race to keep up and accept. It is as if even telephone calls now trick her mind into believing family has been in her room. Our biggest concern now is Joy's desire to "go look for" missing family members. This could result in her wandering off in her quest to find them. She would then check the at-risk box for memory care.

17
Cycles

The "circle of life" has been a theme of many stories and even some movies. Watching this circle unfold in real-time and from opposite sides of the spectrum has been interesting. As we watch the advances our grandson is making, we have noticed how my mom is sliding backward. We look into the eager eyes of our young grandson and see the excitement for the years to come. When we look into Joy's eyes, we see the toll and strain the years have taken, with no glimmer of a future. There are a lot of inverse similarities between the two of them. One is advancing his skills and awareness on a steep learning and growth curve to accomplishments, while the other is rapidly sliding down the slippery slope to incoherency.

We observe this inverse relationship and compare it to either an asymmetric bell curve or beach balls.

As people grow mentally and emotionally, their development has a trajectory moving upward along a curve. This curve continues to elevate until it tapers and plateaus for a period before taking a gradual yet steep decline. While most of us hope for a slow tapering of mental loss, some strive for the normal distribution. Neither of those are options for Joy nor other dementia patients. The mental degradation accelerates alarmingly, while the physical degradation may not. The physicality of a person with Alzheimer's or dementia may be declining at a normal rate, but their mental capacity is declining at an accelerated rate.

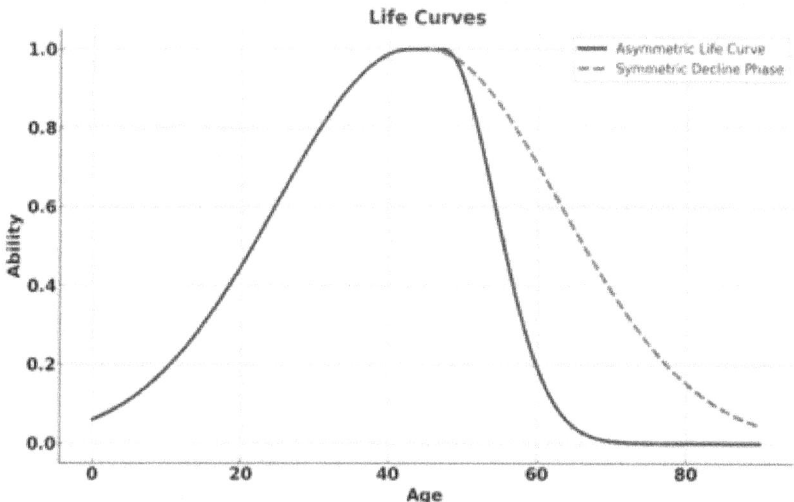

No one's life curve is the same, but the result is an accelerated, irreversible decline.

Another way to look at this is as a beach ball. With every breath of knowledge and experience blown into the new ball, its pliable vinyl skin and vibrant colors swell to take on the bouncy shape everyone enjoys. Filled to capacity, it is ready to maximize its potential, ready for the joys and bumps of life. Over time, the harsh rays of the sun and constant use fade its colors, harden the shell, and thin the skin. The air slowly escapes, no matter how much you try to blow it back up. Likewise, with Alzheimer's, lessons once known leak out, and as the disease progresses, they cannot be recovered or relearned. Over time, they are lost forever. The shrinking, shriveling, once-bright beach ball now occupies space in a box or closet rather than in the center of activity. Seeing it, a tender smile crosses your face as you remember your fun times and memories, knowing it will never be the same.

These are images of how life progresses. Unfortunately, for those with Alzheimer's, the curve is steeper, and the ball degrades faster.

Jan and I have watched the juxtaposition of our grandson at three and Joy at ninety-one. We've observed a similar level of comprehension, independence and dependence, attention span, and ease of distraction. The difference is in their eyes—the bright, eager eyes of our grandson, looking forward to the future; my mom's worn, sad eyes, looking vacantly into the confused past. Our grandson has grown so much in the last year, while Joy has faded an inversely unequal amount.

What this has taught us is that we must appreciate each phase of everyone's life. Over the course of a lifetime, growth and decline are all part of our life stories. Each story is unique, special, and finite. Every day, Jan and I learn to appreciate where everyone is along their life's journey. Realizing our own life's journey is starting to slip and slide down the back side of our own curve, we can only smile at ourselves, knowing our family is nodding their heads as they start to help us when we need it. As we watch with joy as our grandson ascends the path of his life, we watch with sadness as Joy descends the increasingly steep path of Alzheimer's, trying to accept that this is part of her life's journey and helping her along the way.

PART FOUR

We All Need Help

This is a journey no one should do alone. Help and support are available, and you can return the favor.

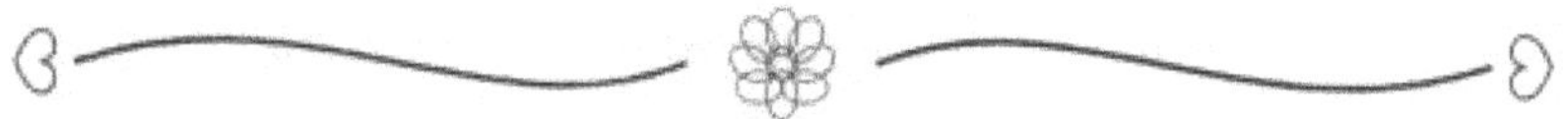

18

Harsh Reality

The First Reality of Alzheimer's is harsh: The person you've loved so long and used to know so well isn't the person you are caring for now. Without sounding too crass, the First Reality means you—the care partner, family member, or friend—are no longer dealing with the person you've known for all these years. You just aren't. Moreover, you will be dealing with someone new almost every day for the rest of their lives. While their memories are being stolen by the disease, yours are being shaken.

As a parent, I had to adjust and grow as my sons grew and matured. I now must do the same, only in reverse, as my mom, Joy, slowly recedes back into her childhood. For some of us, learning how not to treat our 13-year-old like a 5-year-old was hard. It's even harder dealing with an advanced senior who thinks and sometimes acts like a teenager or child. But adjust we must—to where they are in their journey on this narrowing path.

To give care to a loved one with dementia, you need to learn detachment. Without it, you cannot break free of your emotional barriers. With detachment, you will find empathy and patience. You find a way to understand and accept the person you knew is gone.

There is an interesting thrill in discovering the new person. There is also tremendous sadness. You get to choose which you focus on. One gives you the strength to hold up your loved one as well as yourself. It also enables you to hold onto cherished memories and make new ones. The other wears both of you down, crushing a relationship and lifelong memories.

By letting go of the person you once knew, you will find someone new—someone special who is trying their hardest every moment of every day to live with as much dignity as possible. As our loved ones with Alzheimer's lose their memories, continence, confidence, and self-esteem, they are trying their hardest to cope. How much easier is their journey, and ours, when we follow their example and do our best? How much more rewarding is the journey when we strive to make their lives as happy and stress-free as possible every moment we are with them?

I relish the memories of what a special lady Joy was. I rejoice in finding a new special lady every day.

19
Support

Jan and I are grateful to everyone who has listened to and supported us on this journey. Sometimes, simply sharing takes the mystery out of this tortuous path. When doing so, we try to express the sadness, helplessness, uncertainty, and strength that this experience brings. We are finding that dispassionate observations are the best way to recognize change and get ahead of future issues. As difficult and callous as this may sound, it is a way to cope. We are fortunate that many other resources and support teams are available now. I shudder to think what the caregivers of five or ten years ago leaned upon for support.

The following is a list of some books I've read that have helped take some of the uncertainties away:

1. *Creating Moments of Joy Along the Alzheimer's Journey*, by Jolene Brackey
2. *Dementia Caregiver Guide*, by Teepa Snow
3. *Hiding the Stranger in the Mirror: A Detective's Manual for Solving Problems Associated with Alzheimer's Disease and Related Disorders*, by Cameron J. Camp, PhD
4. *I Was Thinking: Unlocking the Door to Successful Conversations with Loved Ones with Cognitive Loss,* by Diana Waugh
5. *In Pursuit of Memory: The Fight Against Alzheimer's*, by Joseph Jebilli
6. *The 36-Hour Day*, by Nancy L. Mace and Peter V. Rabins, MD, MPH
7. *The Caregiver's Guide to Dementia: Practical Advice for Caring for Yourself and Your Loved One*, by Gail Weatherill, RN, CAEd

8. *Understanding the Changing Brain*, by Teepa Snow

We've appreciated books #1, #3, #7, and #8 most on the list. Item #5 was an interesting book, detailing the efforts and discoveries of finding a cure. I'm so glad to know the search continues.

We have joined an Alzheimer's support group at a local retirement community. It is a nice group of people who are all on this journey with a loved one. Interestingly, we are the only ones caring for a parent in the group. All the others are caring for spouses or significant others. The perspectives of caring for a parent and caring for a partner are very different and important to understand. We have an opportunity to escape the burdens and conflicts, and they don't. Their lives are integrally intertwined with their life partner, who is a part of their identity and history. That makes it a lot harder. We also attended a meeting of the Sons and Daughters Caregivers Support Group. Meeting others trying their best to help their parent(s) be comfortable and successful in a difficult time was gratifying. The commonality of these groups is that we are all doing our best to help our loved ones, and we are all at a loss as to what comes next, which is exhausting.

It is important for you to find support so you can support your loved one. The Alzheimer's Organization has resources, an interactive chat room, and significant literature available. Memory care facilities can guide you toward internal and external support groups. These are as valuable as you make them. We've found that the more we open up and express ourselves, the more caring and love we got from the rest of the group.

20

Self-Care Is Critical

Jan and I have been my mother's care partners long enough to realize that we will fight this losing battle for as long as the disease dictates. We also know neither Joy, nor we will be able to mount a successful counterattack. Therefore, Jan and I dig in and adjust to our new reality.

Just as important, we have realized how the disease affects those around us, especially our sons and their wives. We have noticed we withdraw after Joy's phone calls as we try to absorb and rationalize the next Rubicon we've crossed. We have noticed how this withdrawal impacts our sons and their families, and we are constantly working on this, too. They are strong, appreciated support.

Living with Alzheimer's is not for the faint of heart. Nor is being a caregiver to someone with Alzheimer's. Whether you're the primary caregiver or a care partner, it is a full-on, full-time job. It is an obligation and/or something done out of compassion and love—returning the favor for all the years your parent took care of you when you were young or for the times your spouse, sibling, or close friend looked after you when you were sick. The problem is that it is an all-in, all-encompassing commitment laden with emotion and responsibility. Here is the deal: in order to take care of someone with Alzheimer's while also taking care of all your other relationships and responsibilities, you must take care of yourself.

You can try to wink your way through for a while, but you are only kidding yourself. You, everyone, and everything around you can and will be consumed by this disease if you let it. It already has its grip on your loved one, and chances are its hideous tentacles are starting to grab hold of you, too.

Self-care is not being selfish. It is just the opposite. It is the height of compassion and caregiving. You must take care of yourself, health-wise and otherwise, in order to take care of everything else. You must consider and care for not only your loved one with Alzheimer's but also everyone else in your life, including your spouse or significant other, your family, and your friends. Now look in the mirror: "Everyone else" also includes *you*.

Because we don't know if we can or how to prepare Joy, we must prepare ourselves. We will not conquer the disease, but maybe we can calm and conquer anxiety. We make sure to eat right and get enough rest, really rest. We exercise, exercise, exercise—body and mind. We make time to objectively reflect, calming our anxieties and fears. We know this will pass, but until it does, we must be mentally, emotionally, and physically prepared for every known, unknown, and inconceivable unknown. We've also learned that the more you understand, the less you have to fear.

You can never be fully prepared for everything a mind gripped with dementia is going to dish up. But when you prepare yourself as much as possible, you can face whatever you must.

21

Impact on Caregiver

Alzheimer's does not impact only the people afflicted with this hideous disease; it also impacts those associated with them, near and far. It affects those who call, visit, and see the person with Alzheimer's every day. Although the effects on each individual differ, they are unmistakable and memorable.

Jan and I have been asked several times, "How are you doing?" or "How has this changed you?" The answers to such questions will vary for each caregiver, and, frankly, they vary with those of us who walk hand-in-hand as care partners on their loved one's journey down the narrowing, twisted path of Alzheimer's. What affected us at the outset is now a hoped-for situation, knowing we are well past those easier times. Every day is a "new normal," and we must accept it for what it is and embrace who Joy has become and will soon be. To be honest, the new normal is not fun, but then we get our heads around it and remind ourselves that it must be so much harder for Joy.

Our lives have changed and will never be the same, and that is all right. We exercise creative coping and rely upon each other. We make allowances for the way things are.

These days, everything, and we mean *everything*, takes Joy more time. We recognize that simple routine tasks, like getting dressed and eating, take longer and are tiring. Going to doctors' appointments is stressful and exhausting, for all of us. We do not tell Joy when the appointment is; we tell her when we will pick her up and allow 30–45 minutes lead time, knowing the probability of her not remembering is well past 80 percent. We call her a half hour before the pick-up time and are still willing to give even odds that Mom will not be ready. We simply carve out almost half a day for each appointment; and that is all right.

We have found ourselves shackled to our phones. We never know when Joy will call and what emotional trauma or panicked emotion might be affecting her. We take time for our morning, but we know if Joy calls, she is awakening from a delusional nightmare that is very real to her. We abort the workout, meet her in her reality, and talk her through it. Afterward, we are usually too emotionally drained to re-engage in the workout. There is a blessing and a curse to our swim time. On the good hand, our phones are silenced in the locker, and we can let the water slip over us, washing some of the stress off. On the other evil hand, if Joy has called during our swim, there will be at least a half dozen missed calls and voice messages, each getting more panicked, frustrated, and desperate. That reinforces the fact that we almost always have to be in cell coverage and limit our travel and camping to be within about four hours of transit to Joy.

This has given us a whole new appreciation of so many things. This horrid disease has given us a new perspective on patience, acceptance, and tolerance—all of which are probably a great blessing in today's world. We stoically accept our position because we know we cannot change it or change her. All we can control is how we act, respond, and project ourselves to Joy and to each other. We watch and listen to Joy and learn the lessons she teaches us about resiliency, dignity, and perseverance. She did not choose this path any more than we did. The least we can do is help her live her life as best she can.

We recognize, with some despair and trepidation, that if we live long enough, we, too, will succumb to some level of dementia. And so, we try to remain calm, and we willingly apologize for things Joy thinks we've done or said but did not if it eases her anxiety. We trust those who know our situation will understand, and those who don't will quickly figure it out. If they can't, well, that is another story altogether.

We also realize this path has an end. We will be sad when Joy is gone, yet glad when this journey ends. Until then, Joy remains an inspiration in many ways. Like we all do, she seeks relevance in her life and her community.

22

Grandson Calls

Author's Note: This chapter was written by my nephew. It is my pleasure to include his contribution to this book.

It had been far too long since we'd last spoken with Joy. Our schedules have been busy, between my work and the kids' after-school activities. There's also the time difference; Joy is two time zones away, putting her two hours behind us. Then, our winter break RV trip took us to locations with no cell phone coverage. All excuses in the end. In all honesty, writing is thinking, and writing this is highlighting that calling Joy is emotionally exhausting for me, which makes it hard to do. So ... excuses. It had been far too long since we last spoke to my grandmother, Joy, known by her family as "Momo."

Up until six months ago, our phone conversations were on Apple FaceTime. She always seemed to like seeing the kids. But then Joy seemed to be covering the camera so we couldn't see her. Then, our calls to her iPhone went unanswered. So this time I called Momo's landline, steeling myself for uncertainty. She picked up and said hello. Good first step!

"Hi, Momo," I said. A long, awkward pause ensued. I presumed she was striving hard to connect my voice to her memory of my name. Maybe I should have just said who I was when she answered, but I've never done that with her. She has always recognized my voice. So, the long pause was concerning; the rest of the call was even more so.

This was the first time Momo's condition truly expressed itself to us. Until now, she has always been successful at putting up a facade of normalcy on our calls. She's always seemed clear-minded and adept at conversing, albeit with some memory lapses. This time, her voice was shaky and frantic, and she was distraught and hard to follow. She spoke of learning that her husband had passed and that she may have upset everyone because of her struggle to realize this all day. On the other end of the phone, well, I struggled to explain concisely.

It was like the moment a roller coaster starts or a short-distance running race starts—a huge emotional rush, with no choice but to commit to the moment. My brain began rushing with thoughts. *What to do?* My instinct was to comfort her and simmer down the emotion, a tactic works well with the kids. I started with that. Then, just like my kids in the midst of strong emotions, Joy began repeating herself, demonstrating a mental fixation. Her brain seemed stuck on the story. So, like with my kids, my next tactic was distraction.

"How's the weather there?" I asked.

That worked for maybe a half minute. Then we looped back to the story. And it became a bigger loop: comfort, distraction, Grandad's passing, distress, repeat *(Grandad refers to my father and Joy's husband).*

Another loop played out internally within me: rapid decision-making about what to say next, relief when comfort or distraction seemed to take hold, frustration when the reprieve was short-lived, repeat. It wasn't noticeable in the moment, but emotional energy was being burned through rapidly.

Joy provided the out. I couldn't break the cycle. I couldn't leave her like that. But Momo was on a mission. She was already making her way down the hall to tell the front desk that Grandad had passed. Those caretakers have got to be amazing people.

The roller coaster ride was over. It was 8 minutes long, but felt substantially longer.

What now? I wondered.

I turned to my typical evening tasks. I needed action. I needed simple accomplishments: picking up toys and cleaning dishes—easy wins with no emotional baggage. Perfect.

But seriously, what now? Do our calls help Joy? Does she remember them? Does that matter? Should we try to make the cross-country trip to visit, or would that be too stressful for her? Can we hold off until the summer, when our kids are out of school? Or is five months too long to wait? What's best for Joy? If an eight-minute call is a challenge for me, what about my aunt and uncle, who are there with Joy? ... Questions and more questions.

The impact of Alzheimer's doesn't discriminate, it affects everyone, even if the encounter is short.

PART FIVE

Ever-Increasing Changes

Embrace change, don't resist it, because you can't change it.

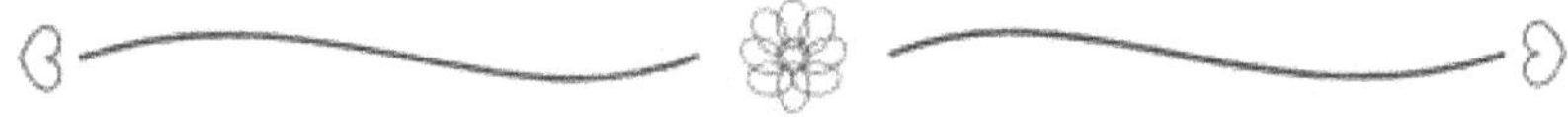

23

Needing More Care

As Joy progresses along her narrowing path, she needs an ever-increasing amount of care and support. Some of this is in the form of physical care, and some is associated with emotional care. The care facility Joy lives in prepares and presents a quarterly care plan for each resident. The plan is based on each individual's needs and then tailored to their individual needs. We find this extremely helpful, and between the plan and a few extra meetings with the team during the quarter, we believe Joy is getting the best care available in our area. We are fortunate. Not everyone overseeing the assisted-living or memory care of someone with Alzheimer's has such an initiative-taking facility, and the responsibility for assessing and adjusting their loved one's needs falls upon them.

We have noticed some very distinct changes in Joy over the last three months, and so has the care team. It would have been easy to attribute the decline to the holidays and/ or the death of Joy's friends, but we are all trying to look past the obvious and objectively assess Joy's current condition. Unfortunately, her decline is very real and probably not reversible. The facility prepares an "acuity score" as part of their program. As the residents decline, their scores drop, indicating more support is needed from the staff. Joy's acuity score dropped from 19 to 11 in the last assessment after being very stable for the previous two quarters.

The new assessment details Joy's need for extra staff time to do many things. She now requires daily queueing and help in dressing. Because Joy has started to forget to go to the dining room to get meals, she has all but one meal delivered each day. She also needs help ensuring she returns to her room after picking up her dinner. She no longer has a clear grasp of where her sanitary products are kept or how to use them. Joy's self-imposed isolation now requires her care team to have one-on-one emotional support up to four times a day a day. This increased support is understandable, given that Joy has been saying her "discussions with Mama and Daddy are so vacant."

Joy now periodically leaves her walker behind and swears she brought it, while it sits in her apartment. This is particularly disturbing in conjunction with her uncertainty about where her apartment might be. We have inserted an AirTag in her walker just in case she does wander off. Yet, if she leaves the walker behind, our proactive safety measure is neutralized. As the weather improves, she may just head out the front door to somewhere she might not know.

Of course, all this extra time, support, and help comes with a cost—a toll taken emotionally, physically, and financially. Fortunately, we are prepared for the latter and are doing our best to manage the others.

This is where Jan and I now find my mom and ourselves. The slippery slope is getting steeper and steeper. Joy calls us three to six times a day now. Usually, she doesn't need anything specific; she's just "reporting in" and/or wanting to know who is in town, where "Mama and Daddy" are, and when supper is. She is perpetually uncertain what time it is, what day it is, when was what, and what is when.

24
Fear and Anxiety

Fear is something that stares you in the face; *anxiety* lurks in the back of your mind. At least, that's what they are when you are mentally competent. When you suffer from dementia, like Alzheimer's, you may not recognize what is real or unreal. Therefore, fear and anxiety become the evil twins you cannot distinguish between. One becomes the other, and they join forces to terrorize your mind and emotions. They torment your dreams and cause panic when you are awake.

Joy's fear and anxiety are now so well blended in her mind that it has become hard for us to differentiate between the two. That is evidently clear when she calls and says the prisoners have escaped and there is rioting down the street. She exclaims that she needs us to come get her and evacuate her to the mainland. We know she is absorbed in the Haitian violence on the news. After she marched down to the front desk with clear intent to ask for a taxi to escape and made several more phone calls to us, she slowly becomes aware it was only the news. There are no Haitian criminals on the loose in Central Oregon. It is the fear in her voice that grips you. The trembling, panicked voice begging us to rescue her lingers long after the call ended.

Then there are the calls and the discussions during Sunday dinner when she is distraught and emotional on a personal level. Those conversations are hard to decipher. Often, she is terrified she has done something wrong, convinced she has offended or hurt someone's feelings.

Joy "Oh, I must have offended your brother and 'mama and daddy' I know I have. I have been in your apartment all afternoon, and no one has come by to see me. I know they are in town. I have talked with them, but I upset them. I did something. They will not come by to see me."

We try to softly explain that it is her apartment, my brother is on the East Coast, and her "mama and daddy" are not in town, and no one is upset.

Joy "Oh, yes, they are. I know it."

We encourage her to call my brother and ask him.

Joy "Oh, no, I couldn't do that. I don't want to bother him. I've already made him mad."

And around the exasperating merry-go-round, we go again.

Joy is dealing with anxiety that turns to fear, which feeds her anxiety, which turns to fear. Unfortunately, she is mentally and emotionally incapable of differentiating between, untangling, or managing those emotions. We do not know why she is fearfully anxious about these mysterious delusional scenarios that cause her so much emotional distress, but she is, and they are real to her. There is no way for us to explain the "unreality" of her reality to her.

The good news is she has no recollection of being distraught, not the next day or after "sobering up," as Joy calls it. Life moves through these horrific episodes and back into her more mundane life of self-imposed isolation and news-watching. The bad news is her agitation is gaining strength and being exhibited publicly. Our concern is her actions may result in her needing to be medicated to help calm her. Another step on the steep, slippery slope of decline.

25
Conscious Subconscious

We all know the feeling: that sensation in the pit of our stomach and in the back of our mind when we know something is right or wrong. That is our subconscious on high alert, silently whispering to us. Sometimes, we listen; sometimes, we do not. We hear it, we feel it, but we rarely talk about it. And we never let it out or allow it to control our actions. For Joy, however, it appears her subconscious is becoming very conscious; she now vocalizes what she hears and feels from deep within.

For a while, she seemed to be enjoying and finally feeling comfortable in her apartment in the assisted living facility. But this has quickly changed. We have watched Joy pack and unpack her belongings several times. Understanding that this action is common for those with Alzheimer's, we did not think much of it. She almost always says she believes her "mama" is coming to take her back home, which is understandable. Her relationship with her mother has been tormenting her.

As we continue to probe gently, however, it is becoming more apparent to us that her subconscious is screaming at her. *This isn't really your home! This isn't really where you want to be! You need to escape!* Her subconscious is manifesting its consciousness verbally and physically. Joy is finding it harder and harder to understand that her room is her apartment. It is no longer a safe haven but a temporary cell.

She calls and pleads, "Come pick me up and take me home. I just want to go upstairs and go to bed."

It is becoming clear that she feels she's not where she belongs and just wants to go "home," but doesn't know where home is anymore.

Joy is still occasionally cognitive enough to know that she is living in an assisted living facility with early-memory care and knows where the memory care wing is located. As we walk past the closed door, she routinely says, "Please don't ever send me to the basement," or "See that door? That is where the needy and really sick live."

There are times at Sunday dinner when she is or becomes clearly confused—wondering where we are, who is visiting, and who is supposed to be dining with us. Then, she will sometimes lean into the table and plead not to be moved to "the basement." Her conscious subconscious is expressing the fear and terror of what she knows, down deep, is her destiny.

Ships seek safe harbors during storms. But Joy's mind will not allow her any respite from the stormy turmoil and confusion. There is no rest, as her slumber is also disturbed. Her days and nights are torn apart and twisted. The earlier torment with the TV news seems so far in the distance now and, ironically, would be welcome. Being able to understand the root of her agitation and talking her through it was so much easier back then. Trying to calm what her disorganized, terrified mind is creating as her subconscious begins to express its control is so much harder and so much more frequent. Once again, we re-learn the hard but simple lesson: meet Joy where Joy is, not where she was, or we want her.

26

More Supervision

Recently, we took Joy to one of her biannual visits with her neurologist. It is always an interesting drive across town and back again. At this point, she is uncertain what kind of doctor a neurologist is and what she should expect. We listen to her constant nervous chatter, unable to interject any answers to her questions.

The results of this last visit will profoundly change her and our lives forever. Her doctor clearly expressed her concern with Joy's confusion of time, location, and awareness of people and places. In her typical Pollyanna way, Joy dismissed the comments and wanted to talk about how much she interacted with people as the Cookie Monster, as if trying to persuade the doctor of her competency and capabilities. The doctor's report was clear: Joy needs "more supervision" and "**would benefit from 24-hour care**."

We completed and returned over a dozen pages of information and forms to the Home Care team to provide more direct care for Joy. We have placed her on the "internal ready list" for memory care. Until an acceptable room is available, she will have someone ready to sit and walk with her as needed. As she declines, she will receive additional services like bathing, dressing, and toileting.

Our concern is that Joy will rebuff the help and not want to be "needy," even if it will help her physically and emotionally. At best, she will be slightly dismissive in her rejection. At worst, she will become agitated and cross. The panacea would be for the care team's patience and compassion to sway Joy into accepting help and enjoying life a little more. It is now sunny and warm, and she needs to walk outside if she can without fear of wandering away.

Joy is now in the queue for a room in memory care, and all our lives are about to be turned upside down; again. As our signatures stare back at us on the waitlist form, there is a bit of remorse and dread. There is a sense we are signing the moral equivalent of a death sentence. At the same time, we feel a sense of reserved relief from the growing fear of her wandering and truncating her isolation. It will be all right. It will be what Joy and we make of it.

The following day, Joy calls, her voice almost giddy with happiness, saying she is now free and a huge weight has been lifted.

"That's great," we say. "What happened?"

"Oh, you know, you put my parents on a plane and sent them home! So now I'm free!" she says joyously.

"That's good," we say. "We're happy for you, Mom."

She calls again that afternoon, saying her mother is back. Her mind is so tormented and tired. And she wants to visit the distant family farm one more time before she dies.

27
New Communication Style

Joy's regression is inversely proportional to her Alzheimer's progression. It is a constant challenge to find ways to communicate clearly with her. As we have mentioned more than once, our goal is to meet Joy where she is, not where she was or where we want her to be. She is where she is at that moment. Frustratingly, the moments can change during the same phone call or face-to-face at dinner.

We are now trying to avoid confusion, conflict, and emotional swings. We had been gently trying to coach her on what was happening in the news or information about the family. We now find that those slight nudges are no longer helpful; in fact, unbeknownst to us, they have sometimes been confusing to her. Earlier in this journey, we desperately tried to remind and guide her while avoiding meaningless confrontations over trivial matters. Now, we just let her talk and try to answer her inquiries without causing confusion. We try just to agree and support. That approach, for now, seems to work reasonably well. So, when she says she is over 100, that's great.

The unintended consequences can be an endless maze to navigate. Although we do our best to agree and support, we sometimes find ourselves in a double-blind, Catch-22 scenario. For example:

Mom "Did you and your brother have a nice time?"

Me "We had a good time."

Mom "Oh, I so much wanted to see you two together. I got cookies from the kitchen to bribe you to come over for dinner."

Or ...

Mom "Did you and your brother have a nice time at dinner?

Me "He's not in town; we didn't have dinner."

Mom "You mean he came all this way and didn't stop by and see either of us?"

Me “He didn’t come to town; he is back East.”

Mom “So, you two had a good time without me while I waited alone in the apartment.”

We opt for the latter. But either way, we often stumble into a hole from which we have a challenging time extricating ourselves.

Mom seems so lonely. Some of this is her own doing, closing herself off in her apartment, and some of it is due to her latest public search for her “mama and daddy.” We have observed some other residents veering to the opposite side of the hall as she walks past, clearly no longer interested in any interaction. Seeing someone go from being so social to now being increasingly ostracized is incredibly sad.

28

Distance Is Hard

The trauma of dementia and Alzheimer's affects not only those afflicted with these diseases but also their caregivers and others who care about their afflicted family member or friend. As hard as it is to be a designated caregiver involved daily, it can be as hard or harder in some ways for those who are far away. Jan and I try to keep that in mind.

We spend a lot of time gathering information on dementia and Alzheimer's, just trying to understand what we are likely to face as Joy regresses. We have a full, ongoing view along this journey, which is both a blessing and a curse wrapped together. We get to observe Joy's changes and swings daily. We witness the ebb and flow of her coherency as well as the swirl of her emotions, fears, and anxieties. Of course, we're also faced with the ever-changing challenge of trying to have light, pleasant conversations with Joy multiple times a day. We sometimes feel as lost as she is because of the frequency of contact and the fluidity of the conversations.

The rest of Joy's family is scattered across the country, which makes personal visits difficult and phone calls a challenge due to time zones. Unfortunately, when they call, they never know where Joy will be emotionally or mentally. They don't know whether she has slipped more since their last interaction with her. While we have become a little desensitized with daily exposure, they get a dose of shock therapy with every call. Witnessing the gradual change afforded by constant contact is, in some ways, so much easier than the major shifts experienced with periodic contact. Thinking you will speak with the same person you did a week or a month ago, only to find someone you almost do not recognize, is nothing short of a shock. The inclination must be to avoid future contact because of concerns about who you will find the next time. It must be heart-wrenching for them to be so far away, unable to help or even to show they care. They must feel helpless, knowing this is out of their control. Conversely, if they could choose, it might be easier to close their eyes and forget Joy's tragedy is happening.

The good news is that Joy's extended family continues to try to reach her. Her older friends have slowly drifted away—some because they are experiencing the same horrid disease, others because they are reluctant to hear Joy this way. And some have passed away. Joy relishes the calls from family and friends and gleefully talks about them for a short while before the memory passes away or is blended with another call or imagined visit. All of the calls are a blessing, and we are sure all her callers are more upset with every week that passes. For Joy, these phone visits with far-away loved ones give her a brief respite from the isolation and sense of loneliness.

29

I'm All Alone

A really sad aspect of how Alzheimer's is affecting Joy is hearing her express her loneliness. Joy was always a little bit of a social butterfly. She would flitter around the dining room and greet everyone, maybe not remembering everyone's names, but greet them, nevertheless. That is, until COVID isolation and Alzheimer's sucked the spirit right out of her. She lost confidence and motivation to be outgoing. Alzheimer's forced a move from an independent living facility to assisted living, after which she ceased to engage with other residents and retreated into her room and the "comfort" of TV news.

With every day of self-imposed isolation comes a greater and greater chance of confusion and depression. When we see Mom in a room with other people, we discretely watch as she seems to wander aimlessly. She is absolutely alone in a crowded room. When approached, she is pleasant and tries to have a superficial conversation. Anything more profound and more thoughtful is now beyond her.

She expressed her concern to us by saying, "I do not like talking to strangers. They might find out how stupid I've become."

This is a moment of clarity in her confusion, leaving another crack in our hearts as she tries so hard to maintain.

In the past several weeks, the facade has fallen, displaying her memory loss to the care team and her neighbors. Joy usually calls us several times a day and almost without fail in mid-afternoon. The calls have become increasingly dark with depression. She does not understand why she has been in her room, alone, all day, and no family has come by or called. She often expresses the sense of having made someone mad and feeling abandoned.

"I'm all alone," she says with exasperation. "So alone." Another crack in our hearts.

A body of research shows a link between depression, hopelessness, and loneliness. Feelings of hopelessness and irrelevancy push those who are feeling alone deeper and deeper into depression. Depression is a state of permanent stress. Anything upsetting or catastrophic, regardless of how minor, releases more stress hormones. This drives the cycle around and deeper, like the twisting of a screw penetrating wood, slow and steady, ever deeper. Sufferers become paralyzed by rigid thinking, deflated by negative emotions, and overwhelmed by uncontrolled hormones. The increased hormones put more stress on the brain's already damaged neurons and receptors, causing more lasting damage.

And so, as the brain deterioration of Alzheimer's steals Joy's episodic memory and her past, so do her isolation, loneliness, and depression begin to kill her mind in another way. This insidious tag team of neurobiological decline and psychological/emotional/social decline may not be one we'll be able to wrestle to the ground.

Maybe the time has come for Joy to move to memory care. Maybe that will provide a way out of or slow down the downward spiral. Or maybe it will inadvertently accelerate it.

PART SIX

Transitions Are Hard

There may never be the perfect moment; sometimes compassion and care prompt the course and timing of action.

30

A Hard Turn on the Narrowing Path

We finally got the phone call we knew was coming and did not necessarily want: the one telling us a lovely room in the memory care unit was available for Joy. We took some deep, hard swallows, talked with the care team, accepted the room, and shed some tears. On the one hand, we sense we are sending Joy downriver. On the other hand, we hope the community will help her become more engaged and livelier. The date has been set, and the anxiety builds.

There are many things to get done, just like with any other move. But this move has to be kept quiet, at least for now. There were transfer papers to sign. Arrangements to be made for the movers: one to move her limited clothes and furnishings from a one-bedroom to a studio apartment, the other to move everything else to storage. We're reading the memory facility's suggested list of items and double-checking our list, while trying to decide which clothes, furnishings, and precious pictures will go to her new room.

We have spent several hours in the memory care area, just hanging out, trying to get a sense of the environment Joy is about to enter. We are fortunate. It is genuinely nice, and the staff seems very friendly. The room is pleasant but small and has a splendid view of the courtyard.

One of the items the care team wants is a biography to post outside Joy's door for the staff, visitors, and residents to read and get to know Joy a little better. This is such a great idea. It helps everyone get to know who is who, and it can be read and re-read as needed:

Joy

Joy was raised on a farm/ranch in West Texas, near El Paso. She is one of eighteen who graduated from Fabens High School. She attended Hockaday finishing school in Dallas and graduated with a

Teaching Degree from Texas Western (now University of Texas at El Paso). After her sons left for college, she earned a Bachelor of Science degree in Library Science from the same university.

Joy loves to walk to the gazebo and watch the TV news. She calls herself an "archivist and news junky."

Joy married Claude in 1952, and they traveled the western United States with his work as a geologist for the first part of their lives together, what she calls her "nomad years." She is a great mother for two sons and a wonderful grandmother to five grandsons and five great-grandchildren. She was the "mom" for her sons' high school cross-country teams and always ready to bake a batch of Vanishing Cookies.

Joy was a substitute teacher and a librarian in many El Paso schools. She proudly served on the Board of Directors of the Lee Moor Children's Home in El Paso. Joy was active in P.E.O., the Presbyterian Church, serving on the Session and loved singing in the choir.

Joy spent almost all her life in the El Paso area, and she loved the desert and the time she spent on the family farm in Fabens, Texas. Joy moved to Bend, Oregon, in 2017 to be closer to family, living in an independent living facility and moving to assisted living in 2022.

That was the easy part.

The hard part will be figuring out a way to tell Joy what is about to happen. We can tell her the truth, or we can follow the dominant conventional practice and fabricate a story. The truth is hard to accept, and the story is hard to maintain. Neither is good. The question is: Which is best for Joy?

The questions swirl in our minds. How do we tell her? How will she take the news? Will she recede further into her shell, get angry, or embrace the situation?

31

The Move … to Hotel California

After extensive discussions with doctors and the care team, we decided to tell Joy the truth about her impending transfer to memory care. We decided to withhold the news until the moving day to prevent her from packing a travel bag and leaving abruptly. Meanwhile, we quietly made our plans and arrangements. We arranged for her neurologist to write a compassionate letter addressed to Joy, explaining she needed twenty-four-hour care for her well-being.

We coordinated with facility staff to move her minimal furniture while Joy was at an audiology appointment. The appointment was genuine, but the extended two-hour wait was planned.

On the return trip, we discussed Joy's increasing care needs with her. We gave her the neurologist's letter. Tears trickled down her face as she read the words "memory care" aloud. I know she understood the words, but probably not the whole meaning. She acted as though she were silently reading the letter again while more tears fell from her eyes. Then she again read out loud, "memory care... "the basement."

In a trembling voice, she protested, "I can't do that. I can't live down there. I just can't."

I touched her hand as I drove.

She read the letter again, more tears streaming. Our words of love, support, confidence, and encouragement seemed to run off of her like her tears were.

Upon arriving back at the facility, she tensed and firmly stated, "I can't and won't live in memory care. I just cannot."

We offered support. "Come on, Mom, you can do this. We can do this."

She started her brave walk into what she felt was the abyss. The abyss of memory care, Dementia, and Alzheimer's were winning the war. With tear-filled eyes as we neared the locked door of the memory care wing, she asked, "Who did I make mad? I am so sorry. I'll apologize. Please."

We reassured her that she had not upset anyone, that this was what Alzheimer's had done to her, and it was not her fault. With our reassurances of love and support, she stepped through the door, her aura filled with fear and anxiety. It felt like the first day of kindergarten.

Joy's new room was bathed in sunlight, with a view of a flower-filled courtyard and a water fountain. Jan had her furniture and selected clothes in their place and arranged family photos on her dresser and end table while Joy was at the audiologist.

We slowly walked to her recliner and sat down for more conversation. She, momentarily, seemed to be coming to terms with her new circumstances but was still understandably apprehensive. We spent what felt like an eternity talking, hugging, and comforting her. Again, we explained in compassionate terms that this was not her fault. It was the disease. It was Alzheimer's. Joy listened and wiped tears from her face. Her sad, tired eyes looked at us, begging us not to do this.

A member of her new care team arrived, greeting her warmly with a nice hug. With this distraction, Jan and I quietly left the room, and the locking door closed behind us. Tears welled up in our eyes as we departed. We were comforted only by the knowledge that Mom is in the right place. She is where she will receive excellent care and pose no risk to herself. She is in the best place for her to live as best she can, but only if she will let herself.

We were reminded of the Eagles' 1977 hit song "Hotel California: "You can check out any time you like. / But you can never leave ...." The next several weeks will be a challenge for us, but especially for Joy. She is confused and in a new community—a community she never wanted to be a part of but is now.

32

Transitions

The first week of Joy's transition from assisted living to memory care has been rough. At this point, if there is a light at the end of the tunnel, it is too small, and the tunnel too long and dark to see, and it may be a train.

Time has come to a virtual standstill—caught somewhere between the delusional world Joy was in and a new reality she cannot figure out. Her body and mind are exhausted, which adds to her confusion and uncertainty. The calls are painful. Pleading for help. Pleading to be with family.

By mid-week, her clarity had improved a little, just a little. By the end of the week, it was like we were starting all over. We talk multiple times every day. We talk and listen. We often mention Alzheimer's—telling her the truth rather than a therapeutic lie—giving her something to blame other than herself, something to be mad at rather than herself and the staff. We give support and understanding while telling her she is where she needs to be and she is in the best possible place—again breaking therapeutic protocol. We listen to her fears and grievances and provide what reassurances and comfort we can.

She was upset with us when we missed several calls while we were out running. The return call started tense, terse, and agitated. She repeated over and over how she could not do this.

Finally, I said, "Mom, look at the palm of your hand.

"That hand brought us into this world.

"That hand held mine and squeezed it with love at the kindergarten door; as you told me, 'You can do this.'

"That hand squeezed mine when I left for college, as you said, 'You can do this.'

"That hand squeezed mine before my wedding, as you said, 'You two can do this.'

"Mom, close your hand and know we are squeezing it and telling you, 'You can do this. We are always here for you. You can do this.'"

Choking back tears, we tried to stabilize our voices while we listened to her sobs. Finally, she said she thinks she can do this and will do the best she can.

Joy, like all of us, wants to feel loved, needed, and not abandoned. She seems to find comfort in our reassurance and empathy. We mix in that she is in the best place and that the disease has done this, not her, which seems to calm her the best.

The transition to memory care takes time, and every transition is different. The memory care team has asked us not to visit for a while, which will be hard. However, it will be harder for Joy to relive all the uncertainty she has already felt over and over until she understands this is our new life, our new reality.

33

Bumpy Road

This last week and a half have been extremely hard for Joy. She has times of slight clarity but longer times of confusion and depression. This bumpy road, with its share of peaks and valleys, is all heading downhill with no prospect of rising back to a level surface. Not even to the elevation she was when she arrived at memory care. We expected the decline but not the tortuous path it is taking.

Joy's mind is playing more tricks on her at an increasing rate than ever before. Her frequent calls are more confused now, with little to no semblance of any reality. We have received some interesting calls over the last several years, but none of them compare to those in the last ten days.

She seems to have grasped the reality of the locked main door at memory care, only to forget and try to open it with all the might of a 91-year-old. She waits for the door to open or tries to slip through if someone lets it close too slowly. She calls and exclaims, "My key will not work!" We explain that her key is to her apartment, not the main door.

Joy "I know that, but my key won't work."

Then, a few days later, the clarity appears as the fog clears.

Joy "I know I'm not permitted to go out without an escort. I know it is for my own safety. I know, but my key just will not work, and it makes me angry."

Then, the fog settles in once again.

The family pictures on her dresser are both a blessing and a curse. She calls and says what a blessing it is to have pictures of loved ones, "But who are some of these people?"

She describes the photo, and we explain. Sometimes, the explanations are accepted, and other times they're met with, "And who belongs to who? And why do I have them?"

Yet, when Joy declares she is packed, quitting her job in memory care, and ready to be picked up, the things she has gathered and placed on the seat of her walker are the family photos.

The last few days have been particularly hard on Joy. While she is becoming more accepting of her new community and living conditions, she has been very depressed about having to plan family funerals. No one has recently passed away; except in her mind and dreams.

She called, declaring that she had made arrangements for her funeral service because she was dying and only had a few weeks to live. As we listened and tried to calm her, she was insistent and gave us details she wanted followed.

In our phone calls over the next few evenings, she kept asking, "How are you holding up?" She believed several family members had been in an accident and died. She expressed that she wanted to arrange and attend the services and said that we should "find your father and my daddy so that they can come too."

All this only to be turned upside down when she was looking at her photographs and exclaimed, "So the man with no fingers and the paratrooper are dead?" The two are one and the same—my father, her late husband of 54 years. One photo is of my dad as a 101st paratrooper during WWII, where he lost several fingers in a jump. The other photo is my dad forty years later. She did not recall his name or who he was, but said, "That's too bad. They were nice."

All I could say was, "Yes, ma'am."

Indeed, Mom, he was a very nice man, and we miss him very much.

34
Genetic Placeholder

At times, Joy's dreams and delusions take her to strange places, in different times, with known and unknown people. As disturbing are the moments of clarity when she expresses her impression of her future.

For Joy, days have become nights and nights, blending in her mind into a confused pattern. Her emotions swing wildly but never toward anything positive. We used to see her having good days and better days. What we now see are bad days and worse ones.

People's identities are blurred in Joy's mind with increasing consistency, and her delusions become increasingly more of her reality. I have been her husband, whom she claims the care team "murdered" and believes she is next. I have been her son, who abandoned her at a cabin, and she now wants to divorce. I have been the ever-supportive little brother, which she never had. And any combination of those people. I am now traveling to West Texas to marry my girlfriend (*shhh* ... don't tell Jan). The roller coaster has few rises, but many tight turns and deep dives.

In the past few days, the darkness has become overwhelming for her. In a semi-lucid state, she takes a deep, exhausted breath and expresses the quiet part aloud:

"There is no getting better, only getting worse."

"I'm just a piece of waste, simply a genetic placeholder waiting for my time to die."

"All I do is occupy space and bother people."

No matter our consolatory words, Joy is hardened in her stance. In a very tangible way, she addresses a gap in our society's perspective of life and end-of-life care. She callously faces the reality of her fate, not of death, but of her extended punishing existence—a meaningless, confused, tortured mind carried around by a strong body refusing to let go of it.

Just as we feel Joy will not see a sunnier side of life, she surprises us. She is worried her parents will not have the money for her to graduate from finishing school, disappointed but more concerned with their financial condition than hers. She walks in a different world every day. Her mind is never turned off and pings around like a ball in a pinball machine, with the flippers working overtime. She needs rest but cannot, seemingly unable to break free from her dreams, day or night.

Nights are days, and days are nights, while Joy's mind swims in a swirl of emotions and tortured memories. We hope to see her roller-coaster ride slow a little and smooth out, if just a little. But do not expect it to do so. We know there is no getting better, only getting worse, and at times so does Joy.

35
First Visits

We've waited patiently and not so patiently for an opportunity to visit Joy. We've been in reasonable contact with the care team and what seems like constant contact with Joy over the last two and a half weeks. At times, we have thought she is accepting her new life, and many more times, we know she has not. Too many times, she has called and said that no one has called her and no one cares. Maybe a visit will assure her. Maybe a visit will rekindle the urge to rebel and the desire to leave. One thing is for sure: we will not know until we try.

During our phone conversation with Joy the night before our planned inaugural visit to her in memory care, she seemed rather calm and in reasonable spirits. We were encouraged. The next morning, however, was a completely different situation. It was like a mind snatcher had taken the calm, pleasant Joy of the evening before and replaced her with an agitated, tormented Joy. We decided to press ahead with a measured amount of anxiety.

Arriving at the memory care door, Jan and I looked at each other, took a deep breath, unlocked the door, and entered the inner sanctum of Clubhouse (the name given to the memory care area to pacify the residents). At the closed split Dutch door of Joy's apartment, we took another deep breath and knocked. We heard the familiar, "Come in," opened the top half of the door, and greeted Joy with the best smiles we could muster. She seemed surprised and very happy. The three of us went to the common area of the Clubhouse and sat together drinking coffee, with Joy fretting about being forced to go to China with her mother and us trying to convince her she didn't have to go. When we finished our coffee, we walked around in the common area and the small courtyard to do something other than talk about her mother.

The visit lasted about an hour. Mom seemed happy we were there and didn't ask to go with us when we left. She and we were feeling pretty good about our first visit and our plans to visit on Mother's Day.

Mother's Day started off poorly, and the next several days were even worse.

On the morning of Mother's Day, there was a breakfast altercation with a resident and the staff. It happens; it is memory care. Joy did not like the situation, and by the time we arrived, she had stuffed her walker with a few things: a slipper, the TV remote, a pair of socks, underwear, and a few small pictures. When we arrived at her door, she was agitated and ready to leave.

She greeted us with, "I am packed. We need to leave. They fight here."

She had received flowers, chocolate, and cookies for Mother's Day. She showed us the gifts and asked what they were for. She had no idea it was Mother's Day and could not grasp the concept, even after numerous staff members mentioned it. We unpacked her walker and helped her get a little more grounded. Despite her confusion over the holiday and upset over the morning skirmish in the dining room, our visit went well overall.

The next several days were more troubling. In Joy's mind, the flowers and sweets implied she was dying, and people were saying goodbye; besides, they cluttered her room. Her calls came at all hours, planning her demise, wishing and pleading for it. At times, she was inconsolable; at other times, she was very stoic and matter-of-fact. She wanted to ensure her parents and husband would be taken care of. She wanted to leave for El Paso, to return home to see those she loved one more time, even though they had already passed. It was heartbreaking.

Joy has continued to be lost in her tormented world. She is still struggling to make sure her parents are cared for after her death, but she is also defiant, wanting desperately not to do anything her mother demands anymore. She wants to be free. Maybe in her clouded mind, freedom is twofold: free from her declining, confused life and free from the torment she believes she faces from her deceased mother.

Our visits will be more frequent, but they will probably not be any less stressful. We hope they help Joy feel a little more secure, and we will pay close attention.

36
The Fishbowl

When we started taking tangible actions to move Joy into memory care, we spent time there and talked with many people whose loved ones were already there. A common thread was, "Just know they will be living in a fishbowl." Little did we know the implications and the impact that reality would have on Joy and on us.

Memory care is a closed society. In Joy's facility, there are thirty-five rooms, which are usually occupied. The residents are all in various stages of mental distress, decline, and dementia, as well as the failing health that comes with their impairment and age. Their exit is locked for their protection, like the glass walls of a fishbowl. They can look out but cannot venture out without an escort. The care staff usually stays uniform, adjusting for days, nights, and weekends. The visitors, so far, are also regulars. We see the same ones when we visit. The scene is set. We are all part of the fishbowl. We are all swimming around and interacting with each other in the random chaos that is memory care.

Within the fishbowl, things just happen. People forget which apartment is theirs and occasionally wander into the wrong room. It is perfectly innocent. They are confused. The confusion is not surprising; all the doors look alike. The residents are easily turned around and continually make simple mistakes. Some have trouble eating and can be disruptive at the family-style dinner table. Some go on "shopping trips" and secure items from others' walkers and open rooms. Items are "relocated" from one resident to another, which is why clothes, phones, and TV remotes are all labeled and why extraordinarily little jewelry is left lying around. The "shopping" is not malicious;" it is just an aspect of their dementia. The staff retrieves the items when the shopper leaves their apartment and appropriately redistributes them.

Personal interaction is fascinating. Everyone, including residents, staff, and visitors, are just fish in the fishbowl. New residents and visitors are new little guppies drawing more attention. Residents cautiously approach newcomers with curiosity and interest. Some come close to get a better look. Others are willing to engage as best they can, even those considered non-verbal, those who converse in their own form of babble speak. Rumors and stories spread quickly in the fishbowl. Each comment, even if heard correctly, is altered just a little and gets increasingly more outlandish and absurd. It is like a version of the children's game, "Pass It On," only significantly out of control.

The residents' world is confined and controlled. The care staff plans activities for those who wish to take part and encourages those who usually do not participate to join in. Joy fits squarely in the latter category. She is uncomfortable with the dementia manifestations of the other residents yet cannot see her own limitations and mental lapses.

Interactions at meals appear to affect Joy the most. This is when there is little room to swim around or away. There can be "altercations" at the dining table as people chaotically move around and occasionally take others' plates. The staff has their hands full.

She reluctantly joins the other residents at the community dining table. It is supposed to be a place and time for people to engage. For Joy, it is a time of high anxiety and discomfort. Her days of flittering around the dining room are long gone. Usually, leaving her meals uneaten, Joy retreats and hides away in the relative safety of her locked apartment.

37
Dreams

We all have dreams. Some of them we remember; some we do not. Some are fun and pleasing, and others can be dark and frightening. We dream of our past, sometimes in mixed collages, and sometimes in almost mystical metaphors. But then we wake up, shake the cobwebs out of our dreamy, sleepy minds, and face the reality of our day.

Some of Joy's dreams are fine, but most are traumatic. And she re-lives them all day long. Some become delusions, a confusing amalgam of memories and waking nightmares that are a disturbing reality for the person experiencing them—and almost as disturbing to those caring for them.

When you are a caregiver for someone in the throes of dementia, it is amazing and alarming how much time and effort goes into this role. It can become all-consuming and occupy every bit of your waking and sleeping consciousness. Sometimes, it fills my mind, posing an unreasonable distraction of thought and planning. But when it invades my sleep, I know it is on the verge of taking control.

I had a dream the other night, and the memory of it still lingers in my mind. I was standing in a doorway, looking into a simple room. There was my Dad, in his early thirties, sitting in a chair. Opposite him, sitting on the seat of her walker, was my mom, frail, tired, and confused, with tears trickling down her cheeks. Dad held her hands with one of his as the other gently stroked her elderly face. There were no smiles, just a sense of love, comfort, and compassion. He turned and looked at me; nodded and gave me a simple smile; then returned his attention to his wife. I awoke, a little startled, and could only mumble to myself. "We are trying, Dad. We are trying our best."

As Jan and I enjoyed our morning coffee, we contemplated the concept of dreams. I thought about how real my dream had been—real enough for me to muster a reply.

We also talked about how real Joy's dreams are for her and how they affect her. We can only imagine their impact on her confused mind. It is hard enough for her to parse hallucinations and delusions from reality during the day. We cannot imagine the impact of how her dreams must torment and absolutely confound her. Joy's nights and naps are not always restful. Her mind cannot stop as it spins out of control between snippets of imagination and her past, present, and current events. Unfortunately, she does not usually wake up with pleasant memories, which is incredibly sad. Her dreams are not her friends. Joy's mind does not reorganize during slumber, as it does for those of sound mind; instead, her mind seems to become even more chaotic.

All we can do when we talk with Joy on the phone or visit is try to help her work through the trauma of the disturbing dreams of her sleeping hours and the trauma of her disturbing delusions during her waking hours.

As you dream tonight, awaken and think about how the dreams of those with dementia and Alzheimer's can be so terrifying, so unsettling. Grant them tremendous latitude as they relive them in real-time with real feelings.

PART SEVEN

Alzheimer's Is Confusing

Watching a child grow is the inverse of witnessing a senior's decline. One is thrilling, the other sad; yet both are critical aspects of life.

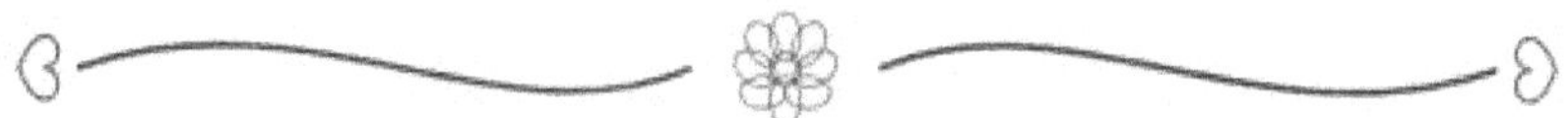

38
Triggers

Jan and I move about our daily lives with Joy in the back of our minds. She is there, always there. We do not talk about it too much, but we both know the phone could erupt at any moment. We also know Joy is losing her ability to manage her cell phone, and if we do not immediately answer when she calls, we will be machine-gunned with rapid-fire calls until we answer. That is our signal that something has impacted her. Something has triggered her, and she needs to talk, and she needs to talk right now.

We never know what has triggered Joy. Sometimes, we don't figure it out for many days; sometimes, we never figure it out. We speak with the care team and with family members of the other residents in an effort to get to the bottom of Joy's emotional state. It is quite an epiphany when we can connect the cause to the effect.

Dreams can trigger behavior, and so can many other things in Joy's daily life. Recently, most of the triggers have been associated with life in the Fishbowl, often comments from other residents or misunderstood events.

For example, a fellow resident with whom Joy tends to dine mentioned she was moving to the East Coast to be closer to family. For the next several weeks, Joy was upset and wanted to move closer to family. She had no specific plan, but she just *had* to move. She could not grasp that we lived nearby, and the rest of her family was scattered across the county. It was immaterial; she was lonely and needed to be closer so more of her family could visit. Joy's dinner companion is still there; through inquiry, we have discovered that she only believes she is moving. It probably does not help when Joy announces that her husband has a new job, and she will be moving soon to join him. The moving loop makes another round through the Fishbowl.

The trigger that seems to affect Joy the most is the physical limitations of some residents at meals. Joy used to be a very compassionate, sympathetic individual who could easily look past the handicaps of others. Unfortunately, she has lost a piece of her character that was so admirable and enduring. Jan and I pensively wait after each meal for the bleak, sullen phone call describing the emotional and physical conditions of these residents. When we visit, Joy not so subtly points them out to us, very much like a first grader pointing out their classmate who is different than others. We ask her to simply be friendly and accepting. We don't have the heart to tell her that, in assisted living, she was the one being pointed out as the odd, vacant woman wandering around looking for a room for her parents.

We have discovered that the primary traumatic trigger of the past, the TV news, does not have the same effect on Joy as it did. She still sits in her recliner, glued to the TV news. But there are no longer the gut-wrenching, panicked calls to evacuate or find shelter based on what she saw on the news. It is almost as if the TV has become essentially background static noise. It seems as though the articles flash past, and the announcers talk too fast for Joy to understand much of anything. At least she is no longer begging to get a car and leave for the airport to escape the riotous mob and devastation anywhere in the world.

We have found value in trying to decipher Joy's triggers. It helps us talk her through the situation and calm her, even if it's just a little. We know the triggers will always be there. New ones will come as old ones leave, and some will stick around like sores for Joy to pick. Now, if we could only figure out the trigger that makes Joy believe Christmas is next month, over and over again.

39
Visits

Visits are essential but can be difficult. As with most things in life, there are positives and negatives to visiting Joy in memory care. The visits range from wonderful to uncomfortable to frustrating, and sometimes all of those at once. Learning to keep things positive and prepare for the negative is our best way to have nice visits. We find short visits are better than long ones. We now visit Joy more frequently, trying to see her at least a few times a week, but we keep the visit relatively short. More, shorter visits are proving to be a much better plan.

Our visits usually follow our morning workouts between Joy's breakfast and lunch. We have found later visits interfere with her resting and can be unsettling for all of us, as she experiences the adverse effect of sundowners in the late afternoon and early evening. Yet, even during morning visits, we can find Joy disoriented, confused, and sometimes agitated if there were any altercations at breakfast. We share a cup of coffee and, weather permitting, take her out of memory care for a walk. This is always done with a bit of trepidation because we never know if she will object to passing through the memory care door and back to her apartment.

Visits can be stressful. Even though we talk with Joy over the phone multiple times each day, not knowing which Joy we will encounter poses uncertainty and a challenge. We have found that no matter the kind of visit, virtual or in person, she is unlikely to recall much of it. Immediately after, she will often comment, "That was nice. Who do they belong to?" Although Joy may not be clear on who she just spoke with, but she knows they were "her people." It is not about how much she remembers; in that moment, she knows she is loved.

Seeing Joy's eyes when we enter her room is very fulfilling. There is a questioning look and then a sparkle, closely followed by a smile. The conversations are always very shallow and usually revolve around a few subjects:

- Something associated with her parents.
- Asking about plans to move closer to family.

We follow along, allowing the conversation to flow as she wants and trying to keep it light and happy. This is when short visits have value, unlike some of our hour-long phone conversations. In person, it is reasonably easy to dance around issues, keep a smile on, touch her hand, and give her a hug.

At the end of the day, Joy, like the rest of us, simply wants to feel loved and cared about, not forgotten and invisible. When we visit, Joy feels good, seen, valued, and loved, even if only for a few moments. It makes it all worthwhile.

However, it is still disquieting for us to see Joy how she is now. It is pretty easy to understand why old friends and other people shy away from reaching out or visiting. It is like watching a terribly slow train wreck, knowing you cannot do anything as the carnage takes place before your eyes. As hard as visits are for us and sometimes for Joy, they tend to be beneficial to Joy, at least for a short time.

40

No OFF Switch

For most of us, we can turn off our minds and relax. We can zone out while watching something inconsequential on the television. We can mindlessly scroll through our various social media. We can lose ourselves in good novels. Best of all, we can relax as we lay down to sleep. Those afflicted with Alzheimer's and other dementias have lost their ability to find and flip their OFF switch. Because it is gone. As a result, their confused minds keep spinning and spinning, like the needle skipping on a scratch of an old record. Again and again flipping back and replaying the segment, over and over again.

Without an OFF switch, the minds of Alzheimer's patients keep running and skipping. They begin to lose sleep and become exhausted. Their fatigue continues the spiral of a confused circular mind. Research has found that deep sleep is essentially a reset button for the brain. It is a cleaning process found to flush the two proteins linked to neurodegeneration (*amyloid-beta* and *tau*) from the brain. Without this flushing, these proteins continue to build inside the neurons and accelerate cognitive degradation. The REM sleep of Alzheimer's patients is not any help, either. For most of us, REM sleep allows us to reorder, reprocess, and dream. For Alzheimer's patients, their dreams are more than likely nightmares, awakening them suddenly and in an even more confusing state. They spend less and less time in both deep sleep and REM sleep, becoming increasingly fatigued and disrupting their circadian rhythm.

For Joy, her paranoia about her "mama" and her thought of moving keep her awake and destroy her sleep. Her sleep is restless and interrupted by thoughts she cannot turn off or put aside. She is increasingly physically exhausted and mentally spent. She calls frequently, and we can hear her physical and mental fatigue in her tired and weak voice. When we hear the exhaustion, we try to keep the calls as short and positive as possible. Conciliatorily, Jan and I encourage her to stretch out and close her eyes, regardless of the time of day.

But Joy's late-night and midnight calls garner a lot more urgency. She wanders around in her tiny room or occasionally ventures into the halls in a panic, looking for her parents. Sometimes, she is lost in time and space, asking why it is dark at ten o'clock in the morning when it's ten o'clock at night; or asking when we are picking her up to travel to Texas or to escape her parents. We listen to the strain in her voice, which prompts us to tell her she must go to bed. If we cannot get her to hang up and try to rest, we know the next day will be long for her and us.

Joy has episodes of sheer panic if we do not answer the phone on her first try. She will robocall every few minutes, leaving increasingly panicked and terrified voice messages. Joy is greatly alarmed if the phone is not answered; sometimes, we simply cannot answer.

There is no OFF switch or even a PAUSE button for Joy's mind. It runs and runs in an infinite figure eight, looping around and around and back again, forward and backward. Joy needs better, more restful sleep, but her mind just will not let her. As hard as we try to lessen the impact of her constantly agitated mind, we watch Joy slowly exhaust herself, physically and mentally, knowing there is little we can do for her. Her facility's caregivers are patient and caring, even on her delusional evening walks.

41

Caregivers

This is a heartfelt thank you to all caregivers.

This is the straightforward reality: During your life, you likely will either:

- Be a caregiver.
- Have been a caregiver.
- Have a caregiver.
- Need a caregiver.
- Or a combination thereof

Whether you become a caregiver willingly or grudgingly, you will find yourself in a remarkably challenging and rewarding position. As Joy's "responsible parties," Jan and I can best describe ourselves as *care coordinators.*

There are many types of care facilities and many reasons to select the one appropriate for your loved one. There is home care, with and without outside nursing care. Private homes offer care and cater to a smaller group of residents. There are more extensive facilities with many residents. These are the choices each "responsible party" needs to assess, and finding the right one for your loved one could take some time. The time spent is worthwhile because they deserve what is best for them.

We picked a larger facility for Joy; her actual caregivers are staff members assigned to memory care. They are the ones who compassionately and patiently care for about thirty-five residents with various states of mental and physical handicaps. Although the residents do their best, you can tell they are somewhere lost in their minds and need the constant, vigilant assistance of caregivers with the knowledge, skill, and patience to help them.

We have silently witnessed the care team perform so many acts of compassion. We have seen them deal with misunderstandings when people sit in the "wrong" chairs for meals. We have seen them cleaning up the inevitable dropped food and silverware while keeping a calm, steady voice and helping those who need more assistance eat their meals. We have watched them guiding the more physically challenged to the TV chairs or to the main table for games and crafts. We've listened while they tried to engage the residents in songs, storytelling, and reading the newspaper headlines. We have watched the slow, deliberate redirection from someone else's room to avoid a conflict. We have watched them prepare to help residents with toileting. These caregivers are people who genuinely care for others.

Their roles, unseen by the curious eyes of the visitors, go well beyond what most of us could imagine. They help with bathing, grooming, and dressing. They have helped Joy keep a little more of her dignity as they deftly usher her back into her room at night after she's wandered from her room in her nightgown. They are attentive and caring. Sometimes, it is not the overt things but the routine observations that matter so much. A few days ago, we were advised that Joy has lost weight since entering memory care. The nurse noted about a 6 percent weight loss and expressed concern, and suggested a protein shake. It is not a big thing, but their attention to Joy is very much appreciated.

Some caregivers specialize in "life enrichment" and coordinate activities for the residents and their families. In Joy's facility, they genuinely care about the whole person and their loved ones who care about them. Joy and we are truly fortunate and very grateful for their care.

Knowing we will all eventually be in the "need a caregiver" category, let's be grateful for both those who accept and choose the caregiver role. We hold a special place in our hearts for all caregivers, whether they've selected that role willingly or begrudgingly.

42
Phone Crutch

Joy still does not interact as much as we had hoped in her new community. But maybe that's because she is on the phone with us for two to four hours every day, and occasionally more.

We were warned. The instructions and suggestions were clearly written on the memory care information sheet: Advise No Personal Cell Phones. But Joy was different, we'd reasoned. She could manage a simple cell phone; surely, she could—right up to the point when she could not. Her cell phone has become less of a communication tool and more of a crutch and an excuse to hide in her room.

We'd realized Joy was beginning to struggle with her cell phone while she was in assisted living. She consistently confused it with the TV remote and the cordless phone. We found she would answer the cordless landline phone but call from the cell phone. We wondered why until it dawned on us that the cell phone had embedded phone numbers, and she had to remember and dial our phone numbers on the cordless. Finding and punching in the numbers in the correct order was becoming an insurmountable task. Nevertheless, she'd felt connected with one of the "three phones" (including the TV remote control she sometimes mistook for a phone).

When Joy moved to memory care, the cordless landline phone disappeared, and the TV remote was labeled accordingly, hoping to avoid confusion. Well, at least that was the plan.

In the months since Joy moved to memory care, her phone has become an unreliable yet indispensable appendage—an unmanageable appendage. We have always tried to keep a "get to" rather than a "have to" perspective. We "get to" answer her calls, and we try to let her express herself as we contemplate the unimaginable and unintelligible. The daily calls have continued without interruption, and the hours have added up. After the twentieth call is answered and the third or fourth hour of her looping phone monologue, our patience is about spent. But, heaven forbid, we do not answer the next call. Joy has an innate ability to call, leave a message, and hit redial on a four-minute cycle until we answer. It is impressive.

In trying to discover why she makes so many calls and for such extended durations, we asked her.

Her answer was straightforward: "I leave my room; I eat my meal. I return to my room and have nothing to do, so I call you."

The life-enrichment team for memory care has many well-planned daily activities. All of them are available for Joy to participate in and hopefully enjoy. We have heard the staff in the background inviting her to join the group activities.

Joy's answer: "No, thank you. I'm on the phone with my family."

From when Joy wakes up until she closes the day, accounting for her meal and rest times, we figure she has about four to five hours to fill. It is not a coincidence that much of that time is spent on the phone with us. Joy is clearly using the phone as a crutch to avoid interaction with other residents and staff in memory care. We have inquired, and the staff has confirmed they believe Joy is avoiding group activities and is using phone calls as a crutch not to engage. They strongly encourage us to take the phone, even for a few days, to see what happens. Joy needs to be involved in her new community and their activities, but she also needs a way to reach out to family and not feel abandoned and isolated.

Unfortunately, technology is no longer Joy's friend and has become a nemesis out to get her. It is not an operator error; it is undoubtedly the phone "acting up." Joy grew up with party-line phones, when phone numbers were three or four digits at most, and someone else was always on the line listening and willing to help. The process of working the phone is now unfathomably complicated for Joy. Letting her keep it and somehow manage her call time will not solve the exasperating frustration of trying to use the phone or trying to use the TV remote as a phone.

So, we are considering the staff's suggestion to "temporarily" remove Joy's phone. Maybe then she will respond to her community, or maybe not. But we think we need to find out.

43
Personal Stigma

We think we are on the right track, and Joy calls:

Mom "Hi. I was getting organized. Can you tell me what day in March it is?"

Me "Um, Mom, we're sorry, but it is July; July Fourth."

Mom "Oh, it can't be! It just can't be. I've lost so many months, so much time. I'm so confused."

Let's be honest: there is a stigma with Alzheimer's, dementia, and other neurobiological illnesses. You can see it. You can feel it. And guess what? So can those who are afflicted. They feel and hear your discomfort. They notice your avoidance and distancing. Unfortunately, they also usually suffer from *anosognosia* (the inability to recognize their mental/behavioral disorder) to a greater degree than others. They suffer from a level of denial and try to hide their affliction for as long as they can. This is true for Joy as well.

Persona is Latin for the English word *mask*, and we are all actors in the theater of life. Which act of the performance are you in? There are many unique things about being "the person" for an Alzheimer's patient; you get to hear what they are trying to hide but what everyone knows. For a very long time, like most of us, Joy has had a couple of personas. She has one for public consumption and the other privately reserved one for her special people. This has only been enhanced as her Alzheimer's has advanced. She will tell us stories on phone calls:

Mom "I'm being deployed very soon and will be out of touch."

Me "Oh really, where and when are you going?"

Mom "I don't know, but it will be very soon. Mama can't go to war anymore, so I have to take her place."

Me "Okay, well, you be safe."

Mom "Oh, I will, but don't tell the staff. I know it sounds crazy, and they think I'm the only sane one here."

Me "Okay, we won't tell."

She will describe the manners of her dining mates in great detail as she struggles with her small piece of pizza. Joy, like most of us, can see the problems others have, but she cannot, or will not, see her own. She will say she is "diminishing," but in the next breath, she will boast about volunteering to help with the night shift—seemingly believing she is more than qualified and capable of aiding the staff.

As Joy shields herself from herself, it is both interesting and sad to observe the shields of others, too. There is a sign-in log at the memory care locked door. Visitors are asked to identify themselves, their in/out times, and who they visit for tracing purposes. A key request is to specify **who** is being visited. We jot down Joy's name and then flip through the log-in sheets. We make a mental note that less than two in twenty have identified who they are visiting. All others have written the room number rather than the name of the loved one they've come to see. Even for those visiting memory care, it seems that Alzheimer's and dementia still carry an impactful stigma. We wonder what prevents them from simply noting "who" they're visiting in memory care. It is not like it's a secret. On every door of every room is the name, their photograph, and a lovely biography of the resident living there. As we enter the Fishbowl, we wonder how, if those visiting cannot avoid the stigma of mental illness, how will those afflicted ever be able to?

We are Joy's "peeps." We are privy to her private thoughts like no one else. We hear and see the bad and the ugly but very seldom the good. Joy reserves her "everything is fine, and I'm alright" external persona for others. We see the silent part. But the silent part— *shhhh,* do not tell is that Joy has Alzheimer's, and she is losing her memory and her mind—is to remain hidden, behind closed doors, between us caregivers and our loved ones suffering from these "unspeakable" mental disorders.

On second thought, please do tell. Say it out loud. Please take a deep breath and say it again and again. It was hard to talk about Dad's cancer, but we did. The world is more accepting and supportive of physical illnesses like cancer. Maybe the more we discuss mental illness and dementia, the bolder and broader the support for its research will become. Perhaps the stigma will fade away if society embraces those in need of mental health care as people in need of health care.

44
No Net

It's been over a week since Joy's cell phone was removed from the death grip of her old fingers. She hasn't been without a phone during this time. She has access to a community phone, affectionately called the "Family Phone," in the open area of the memory care unit. This phone is for the use of all residents to call out and for family members to call in. We have left her access to the Family Phone to the discretion of the care team. As a result, we can talk with and call Joy at least once a day. However, the duration of the calls is limited and managed.

The staff highly supports our decision to remove Joy's "safety net" cell phone. Without it, they could see a part of her that she was hiding. With this fuller perspective of Joy, they can better help her. It forces her to step out of her apartment and begin to become a member of her community. Whether she knows it or not, her safety net is much bigger and stronger without her cell phone than it is with it.

The daily phone calls we get are still bothersome and confusing. They are focused on her fixation and anxiety with her mother and with her asking why "your father" hasn't called. Although she often talks about how "isolated" She is, we know she is more socially engaged than before. Her claims of "isolation" may mean she cannot make countless, never-ending calls, and that transition is difficult.

Joy no longer talks much about anything related to memory care or the other residents. We believe she isn't encouraged to take the Family Phone to her apartment. That forces her to call from a communal area, which, interestingly, stifles most of those topics. We have discovered that she no longer wants to have any semblance of a conversation, just a monologue. Calls are limited to about a half hour, and during that time, we find it much easier to mute ourselves and let her vent. Her determination to explain her delusional anxiety of the moment buries and blurs any attempt we might make at dialogue.

Joy is more easily distracted than ever before. We had a challenging conversation late one afternoon. She slipped into her "I don't have" routine, and it didn't go well.

"I don't have any money. I don't have a credit card. I don't have any stamps. I don't have any Christmas cards. I don't even have a car to get anything. I don't have..."

After about 20 minutes, we interrupted her and asked if she would like to have dinner with us. Her initial silence was disturbing. She stammered a little as if she were having to mentally shift gears, and then she welcomed the invitation.

She was waiting for us. As we approached the locked security door, we saw her fingers pressing against the small window and then her face peering out. She seemed surprised to see us, which was surprising to us. Her clear anxiety seemed to abate.

And then: "Where are Mama and Daddy? I was expecting them, not you. I'm so relieved it's you."

Dinner took on an entirely different tone than we had anticipated. In the course of an hour, Joy had forgotten our tense call. Her anxiety quickly vaporized, but she repeatedly asked where her parents were. It was like a few electrical breakers had been switched on and off. What had happened never did, and what was expected never will. But she won't remember.

45

Free at Last

We find ourselves looking for the small things to smile about because there are so few big things to smile about anymore. Joy seems calmer over the last week. She seems less agitated and a little more relaxed. It may be our imagination, but by not having her cell phone, the endless frustration of her trying to make it work is an irritation removed. Joy still mentions her desire to have a phone, but her insistence and dependence seem to have abated, at least for now.

We're concerned about Joy's lack of social engagement and interaction. She used to be so social, but she isn't social anymore. In the interest of trying to help her, we started thinking about aspects of depression. Depression can be a symptom of Alzheimer's, and understandably so. A recent online post highlighted some interesting points. People suffering from depression can typically exhibit the following:

- Their room is their safe place, and they feel threatened and insecure when they leave. CHECK!
- They spend hours doing nothing, waiting for any motivation to come their way. CHECK!
- They can't fall asleep or have restless, sporadic sleep, even when exhausted. CHECK!
- They procrastinate because simple tasks are seen as almost impossible. CHECK!
- They pretend to be busy, with anything, to avoid conversations and personal interactions. Joy's tool of choice was her cell phone. CHECK! and CHECK!

Alzheimer's never takes a day off. It is constant and exhausting. We wonder whether Joy, along with dealing with her memory loss, is also struggling through her version of depression.

There are lighter moments that make us giggle. Every time we visit and go for a walk or go out for a pizza, without fail, Joy asks how she can get one of the "magic keys" to open the locked door of memory care. As the door opens, she exhales profoundly and loudly proclaims, "Free at last," like a 1960s civil rights advocate. As we walk past the kitchen, the staff warmly greets her, and she loudly proclaims that they were the ones who helped her be the Cookie Monster. And smiles come to every face. Some memories are still made and are happy. Stepping out the front door, Joy again sighs deeply and loudly proclaims, "Free at last!" She takes a deep breath and says she hasn't been free in months. We tell her that it is shocking, but we're glad she is free now, as we start our slow, methodical walk around the building, which she won't remember by day's end.

It is interesting to see what reactions result from actions. Escorting Joy out of memory care is always interesting and usually adds lightness to her day and ours.

46

Myths and Confabulations

There are a lot of myths and misunderstandings swirling around Alzheimer's, dementia, and mental illness in general. That is understandable, as those who are supposedly "sane" are trying to explain those who are deemed "insane." Yet, as in most things, perspective is so critical. Would we consider people with dementia, Alzheimer's, or another mental illness as "crazy" if we could see the world through their eyes? From our "sane" perspective, their actions may seem disturbing, but they are probably perfectly reasonable from their point of view.

There are other generally accepted concepts that seem perfectly reasonable to us, the so-called "sane," but may not be. The idea is propagated that once those with Alzheimer's or dementia have forgotten something, they can't recall or relearn it. Nor, supposedly, can they learn something new. Really? Ask yourself, what is learning?

Jan and I fell into that perspective as we watched Joy muddle her memories and confuse the words of her once robust vocabulary. Yet, Joy continues to learn and demonstrates she can. No, she can no longer demonstrate mastery of a cell phone, and yes, she struggles with how to use her metal room key, but she still learns. Joy has been in memory care for a little over three months. She was moved without any warning or preparation. Yet, in this time frame, she has learned which room is hers and where it is. She has learned the faces, and most of the unique idiosyncrasies of other members of her closed community. She has learned the community schedule and interesting social norms. She has even bragged about giving "presentations" at the dining table on how she uses her room key and how the zipper on her vest works. She seemed so proud when she told the story.

We've also noticed an increase in delusions and confusion when Joy mentions a disrupted night's sleep. After some research, we read several articles discussing how memories are imprinted in the brain. One in particular, "*How the Brain Decides What to Remember*" by Y. Saplakoghu (wired.com), referenced the important work Dr. G. Buzsaki of NYU has done on the subject of memory building. Simply, storing memories requires each of us to drop into a deep-sleep state. That is when the electrical ripples are pulsed, and memories are stored. We contacted Dr. Buzsaki with our observation. To our delight, he quickly responded and confirmed what we thought. He wrote:

"The hippocampal sharp wave ripples are altered in Alzheimer's patients. In addition, epileptiform events develop from sharp wave ripples which hijack the beneficial effects of those physiological patterns. Many Alzheimer's patients are treated prophylactically ... for this reason."

Episodic memory has been mentioned before in this book. We now recognize that altered sleep patterns can induce even more confusion. So, it isn't that Joy is making up stories when she expresses panic and paranoia about her mother. It is a memory error, a *confabulation.* To Joy, her hallucinations are real. Her delusions about being controlled and kidnapped by her mother are dangerously accentuated, putting her into a panicked paranoia and affecting her digestive health. She isn't lying. To her, this is all very real. If we could see things through Joy's mind, we might be terrified, too.

We genuinely think Joy can still learn, even though she seems to read the words with little to no apparent comprehension. She has learned to survive in her new society. Her confabulations are not lies, but rather just a swirl of confused, interlinked memories.

We hope Joy can relax and get some better, deeper sleep, because we now know that will help. Remember, we are all a little "crazy." Maybe we should try to understand theirs.

47

I Don't Have ...

We all know people who have the greatest intentions of accomplishing much but accomplish little. They always have a plethora of excuses—of course, none of them are their fault. They always seem to find something, anything, they need to have before they can get started. We now find Joy with the same frame of mind.

Joy has ideas of things she wants to accomplish but always finds something she needs before she can start. In her past, she was much more focused and accomplished. She didn't make excuses for not getting things done. She just got things done. Now, as a result of Alzheimer's, there seem to be so many hurdles, roadblocks, and things she must have before she can even start simple tasks.

Joy's mind journey now latches onto a few recurring themes:

- The paranoia of being forced by her deceased mother, "Mama," to take a trip with or to help her.
- The location and security of her prized journals.
- Her isolation.
- The compulsion to send Christmas cards.

These themes are repeated in a never-ending infinite loop during the course of each day and week. Each of these themes is given its proper place and importance and very rarely interferes with the others.

It is with the unyielding pursuit of Christmas cards that Joy's desire to have everything in place before taking any action is the most dramatic. In the past, Joy took considerable pride in her Christmas cards and letters. They were quite the production. Her full-page draft letter was sent to everyone in the family so that they could edit their portion “for accuracy.” She would then look through her 3” x 5” index card box. This wasn’t any ordinary card catalog. The updated address and any notes of deaths, births, weddings, or divorces were on one side. On the flip side, Joy would record the year she sent the card and note if there had been a reply or not. She did this for many years. She was, to say the least, methodical.

But now, Joy becomes anxious and worries about her Christmas cards. This year, it started in March, and with each round of anxious looping, it goes like this:

Joy “I don’t have pretty paper,” with exasperation.

We gathered some pretty Christmas paper from years past and gave them to her. But no draft of the letter was prepared.

Joy “I don’t have stamps.”

We gave her a roll of stamps, which are now lost somewhere in her room.

Joy “I don’t have a typewriter.”

We offered to type anything she wrote for her to proofread and edit, but there is still no draft letter.

Joy “I don’t have my card file.”

We gave her a list of family and close, still-living friends’ addresses, yet there is no draft letter.

Joy “I don’t have any money or a credit card to order anything. I don’t even have a car to go shopping for Christmas.” (For which we all are eternally grateful.)

One excuse after another regarding actions that are out of her control. Writing Christmas cards, the one thing she could do, something she looked forward to and relished doing, she can not do anymore. She’s lost the ability to recall and compose. We encourage her to try to write some ideas for her letter but know the whole subject weighs on her. Our attempt at encouragement is greeted with, “Don’t lecture me.” As a result, Joy’s level of frustration increases, and the conversations continue to swirl down the drain. We understand all the other “I don’t haves” are really a rouse to cover the real issue: she just can’t write the letter. Like most things, the joy of Christmas cards and letters has become a chore, a duty that Joy feels compelled to do and simply cannot.

48

Split Personality

The journey we walk with Joy in Alzheimer's isn't a straight path. It is a winding, twisted, narrowing path with no guardrails. There is barely room for one guardrail, but we still try to squeeze on and lend a hand. Joy is slipping farther from the world of reality and deeper into the world of her now-contorted past.

Joy's frustration and isolation are beginning to fundamentally change her personality—or at least the persona she presents to us. We believe the Joy the staff sees is different from the Joy we see. We've seen how Joy can display at least two personalities, like turning a light switch on and off. Recently, those different realities and personalities are beginning to blend together more, but they are still present.

The liberation of her cell phone has yielded intriguing results and insights. We always knew Joy had an act she could put on briefly for the staff and visitors. We were the ones she reserved her darker side and complaints for. The staff knew the Joy she wanted them to for a long time. The Joy who was busy on the phone. The Joy watching TV news to "stay informed." But then she began to slip, and the actual degree of how far she'd slid down the Alzheimer's path began to show. She could still hide a lot by picking up her phone, calling us, and hiding in her room. But with her cell phone gone, Joy has started to engage with the memory care team and with other residents in a whole new way. The persona of Joy they're now meeting looks and sounds a lot like the Joy that we, unfortunately, hear and see most of the time.

The staff now dials the "family phone" for her. When we answer, there is usually a short window when we can hear both Joy and the staff member. Listening to Joy's interaction with the staff is a constant source of amusement and bewilderment. She is calm and pleasant with a cheerful voice. Then she says hello to us, and the switch is flipped.

She's unhappy and distraught. She is afraid, upset, and anguished. She starts in on one of the four main topics, her list of "I don't haves..." She simply wants to vent. To express her darkest thoughts. To deliver a monologue, without suggestions or questions or other semblance of dialogue with us. Until she relinquished her cell phone, the staff saw some of this, but not as much as we would have hoped. They now get to see more than we do. As a result, Joy is getting better care, which is good.

The nurse has told us Joy is in a transition—a transition between our world and the exclusive world of her inner mind. The nurse tells us it is heartbreaking to watch the faces of residents as they momentarily come out of their fog and realize how lost they really are. We have seen that face. The eyes clear and focus momentarily, and as quickly as they do, they can fog over. Joy calls people who aren't clear-minded and present "vacant." She, too, would now be labeled "vacant." But it isn't the correct term. Joy is very clear in what she wants, from her perspective. Even when she seems to be in her "babble speak" mode. Yet, Joy still refers to many of her fellow residents in memory care as "vacant." From our perspective, based on our talks, calls, walks, and dinners with Joy, she is missing more than she is present. But she can still put on one helluva show for a moment or two.

PART EIGHT

The Hardest Decision

Some of your decisions might bring comfort while accelerating death; prepare yourself.

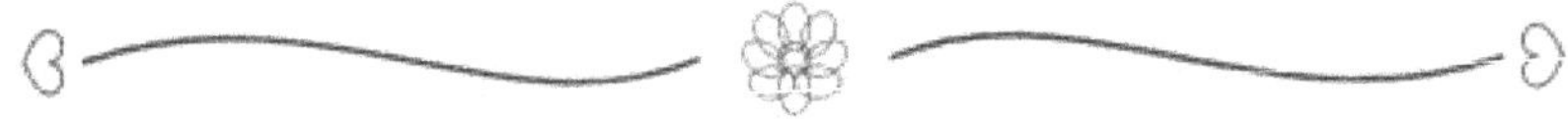

49

The Final Fall

We got another call. The call we'd hoped we had evaded but expected and dreaded: Joy took another tumble, a bad one. We knew there was always a chance of her falling again with potentially catastrophic consequences. In the past five years, she has tripped or lost her balance and fallen several times—each involving a ride to the emergency room. Earlier falls resulted in a broken shoulder and concussions. As traumatic as those falls were, this one will impact Joy's journey profoundly. This time, she broke the femur neck at the hip, bruised her knee, and ripped a swath of her paper-thin skin off her forearm. Mom was being who she is, helping another resident get in and out of a chair, when she lost her balance and fell.

Looking at her now as she lies in a progressive-care hospital room, her pale skin drawn and her pink lips quivering a little, I realize she doesn't grasp what impact this will have on her life.

The hospital staff come and go repeatedly and always ask her why she is there and when she was born. Joy struggles with any reply. She knows her hip hurts but cannot articulate why. She doesn't understand her strange and unfamiliar surroundings. Her confusion is reaching all new heights, and her eyes have a distant glaze. With every question, she turns toward us with pleading eyes for help.

Joy's surgery went well, but the road ahead will be fraught with more unknowns than knowns. On her journey, we were hoping to avoid the intersection of Alzheimer's and a broken hip. This crossroad must be confusing and terrifying all at the same time. She is experiencing general confusion, paranoia, and delusions with a healthy dose of pain to keep it real. Statistically, the odds are now squarely against Joy. She has already shown an increased cognitive decline, delirium, and paranoia. Pain management is an issue because

Alzheimer's patients have a decreased ability to feel pain, identify sources, and have trouble communicating both. Her appetite is non-existent. It is hard to convince her to eat and drink. But those are the simple things.

Elderly (90+ years) Alzheimer's patients recovering from hip surgery have less than a 15 percent probability of regaining full mobility. The odds are against Joy walking again. She has never before faced this type of difficult, painful physical challenge. She's got one now, and how she responds to rehabilitation will dictate her results. The mortality rate for someone in Joy's condition is just as bleak, if not darker. In Joy's situation, the six-month mortality rate is exceeds 80 percent.

Statistics and probabilities are just guideline numbers to help ensure we are aware of the likelihood. This has been and will be a rough patch in our journey with Joy. We sit by her hospital bed and calm some of her paranoia, and we are relieved as she relaxes and drifts off into a restless nap. Her mouth is slightly agape, her hair is matted and partially combed, and her eyelids twitch somewhat. She replies aloud to an unheard question in her mind, and drifts back off to sleep. We know this could be the beginning of the end and want to do what we can to make it special and calm.

50

Physical Therapy Options

We are trying to figure out the next step—what type, duration, and location of treatment and care Joy will now receive. The quality of care isn't the issue; the biggest problem is maneuvering through the administrative bureaucracy.

Joy's stay at the hospital lasted six days. She moved from the emergency room to progressive care and surgery and finally onto the orthopedic floor of the hospital. The staff has been caring and thoughtful as well as very understanding of Joy's cognitive decline. They've followed along with her stories of being in New Mexico, the restless sleep outbursts, her introducing me as her brother, her delusions of listening to concerts in Mexico, and her paranoia that all of this was a ruse to get more money for the government. In these few days, it is apparent her cognitive decline is accelerating because of her trauma.

A flurry of discussions focused on getting Joy the best medical support possible following her discharge. There are many potential issues related to her fall and surgery. Beyond wound management and physical therapy, her dementia also needs to be considered. It became clear we had only two options: (1) a transitional facility and (2) a return to her memory care apartment.

Several opinions were expressed that memory patients can't follow directions well enough to benefit from physical therapy. (Obviously, they haven't read Chapter 46, Myths and Confabulations.) These voices advocated for a return to the familiar surroundings of memory care with contracted special in-home care. In the transitional facility, Joy would get *daily* physical and occupational therapy and wound care. At memory care, she would get physical therapy and wound care roughly three times a week.

Because Joy was in the hospital for more than three days, Medicare would cover a period in a transitional facility, but there would be limited coverage for in-home care at her apartment. We felt the increased repetitive sessions in the transitional facility would benefit Joy. Daily practice could give her the best chance to walk again. In the transitional facility, she would also be closely monitored for all the other possible side effects of the fall and surgery.

Listening to the myriad opinions, we decided. Six days after her fall, Joy moved to a transitional care facility.

Joy's wounds go beyond her broken femur and the massive skin tear on her left forearm. Her fragile skin tore so quickly, and the large, exposed wound will be so hard to heal. Her blood thinning medication resulted in significant bruising and blood loss in surgery. Her left leg and hip are terribly swollen, as the trapped fluids find weak points and continually ooze. Joy comments about the pain in her left leg but doesn't claim it excruciating. Pain management is complex with a patient who can't really feel pain or discuss it with clarity.

The real struggle is her mind. Joy hasn't had a clear moment in a week. She is totally lost in her memories, and they are more scrambled than ever. Studies are showing that post-anesthesia, there can be an irreversible cognitive decline. We think we are witnessing that very thing. While we try to get the physical part of Joy well, we face the reality she will always have difficulty walking, if she's ever able to walk again. There is also the very real probability that she will not have another cognitive moment.

We watch as she refuses to eat or drink much of anything. She doesn't seem to want the distraction of the TV, so she sits silently, lost in her confused mind. We sit by her bed, and we're there to encourage her during her meals and training. Life just got a lot harder for Joy.

51

Day by Day and PTSD

Moving to transitional care has proven to be more traumatic than expected, but we should have expected it. The last several days blend together without distinguishable breaks. Every morning, we park the camper near Joy's transitional care facility and spend the morning trying to encourage her to eat and drink and watching her drift off to sleep. Slipping out the curtained partition, we escape to the solitude of the camper for a bit of lunch and a quick, quiet rest. Returning to Joy's room, we usually find her in a very disturbed state.

Joy is fully embroiled in the darkness of an evil trifecta. She is suffering from advanced Alzheimer's, trauma of a broken femur and surgery, and now a case of post-traumatic stress disorder (PTSD). We sit with her to calm her or take her outside in her wheelchair for some fresh air and distraction. Returning her to her room, she dozes off, and we return home. We get some exercise and some downtime and prepare to start all over again the next day.

Joy has more intense delusional events as she suffers through the discomfort and weakness of her condition. We try to meet her where she is while also trying to understand the triggers. We arrived at the facility to find her distraught, claiming that the staff was blaming her for an unknown man's death. That she has driven to and just returned from Central Texas and New Mexico. That she has joined the army, and anything she does is part of a government conspiracy to trap and enslave people. That her mother allowed her to be physically assaulted in a trailer in New Mexico, and she is now one of the victims. That she has been diagnosed with breast cancer, and her breakfast cinnamon bun is food for those about to have chemo and die. We never know what we will hear, where she will be, or frankly, how to react other than to try to calm her and let her express herself.

Joy is totally disoriented, which creates some significant safety concerns. The operating protocols of transitional care facilities don't allow them to use beds with full-length side rails, fall alarms, or any form of constraint. We fully expected Joy to forget where she was and why and for her to have another fall getting out of bed. Our expectations were realized during the third evening. Joy, in confusion, tried to get out of bed and fell onto the hardwood floor. The care team called, and we returned to the facility to help calm a severely agitated and fragile woman. After an hour, we finally convinced her to go back to bed, and we sat with her until she was asleep. We hope the fall won't add to her complications, but we know there is a chance it might.

It is sad to watch my mom in physical pain and such mental and emotional disarray. Her wounds are dressed three to four times a day, which is the care she needs. The staff is caring, but they also struggle with how best to communicate with Joy in her delusional world. The lack of nutrition and fluids is another concern.

52
Slipping

Joy has struggled since the second fall. She doesn't seem to be in significantly more pain, but her mood is darker. Her appetite is non-existent. Her physical and occupational therapy efforts have decreased in line with her appetite. Over a four-day period, she has, at best, picked at her food or, more commonly, ignored it altogether. She takes a few sips of coffee or drinks only when taking her medication and then only enough to swallow the pills. She claims to be too weak to push herself up onto her two-wheel walker during PT and to try to push her wheelchair. She rejects efforts to take her outside.

We are there to greet her every morning. She is deeper into herself, describing conspiracy theories of corruption and entrapment, and generally in a much darker disposition. Joy dismisses her meals after about a half-hour of them being placed before her. She says she is tired. She is helped back into bed and falls into a disturbed sleep. We sit and watch Joy's hands shake, and her lips quiver before her mouth drops open. She talks to the people in her dreams and awakens with a start, only to repeat the cycle.

We have lengthy, thoughtful, complex discussions with the care team, trying to determine what is best for Joy. Her lack of nutrition is terrifying and not sustainable. We cannot determine whether Joy is giving up or her body is shutting down. Either way, she is slipping, slipping away. Joy's care directive is unambiguous. She doesn't want any heroics for survival—no resuscitation, no intubation, no CPR, no feeding tube, no feeding assistance ... as she would say, "no nothing."

We bring in a palliative care doctor to give an assessment and discuss options. As we talk, sitting next to Joy, watching as she goes through her "sleep cycle," he calmly, empathically says, "That is what coming death looks like." He advises we arrange for hospice care and return Joy to her memory care apartment. We understand, but Joy has a prearranged, post-surgery orthopedic follow-up later in the day. The palliative care doctor asks why we are going. We talk about the two paths we are upon. One path plans for physical recovery, allowing Joy to be somewhat ambulatory until her mind and/or body fails. The other path prepares her and us for her end of life. We must walk down these paths concurrently until it is obvious one is no longer an option.

So, we proceeded to the orthopedic follow-up and heard what we really didn't want or expect to hear. The main pin/rod holding Joy's femur in place has dislodged, requiring surgical repair. Joy doesn't understand what her weekend fall has yielded, and we aren't sure we fully understand either.

Joy doesn't return to the transitional facility; instead, she is re-admitted to the hospital. We engage with a team of doctors, including the emergency room physician, an orthopedic surgeon, an internist, and another palliative care physician. They understand the conundrum and the almost impossible decision we must make. They explain that if the damage isn't repaired, the femur will never heal, and Joy will be in severe chronic pain with every move forever.

Meanwhile, Joy is lying on the ER gurney with IV tubes in her frail, thin arms. Her horribly bruised left leg peeks out from the warming blankets. Her unfocused eyes look around, and with a clear voice, she says she's happy to be here and smiles.

We decide we cannot deny her the chance, however slim, of eventually being pain-free and ambulatory, for whatever time she does have left. She is moved to the orthopedic wing and scheduled for her next round of surgery.

53

Following Joy's Lead

Joy took our hands and walked us through the "un-amusement" park, and then she stepped into a lonely roller coaster car. We climbed into the car behind her as it jerked to a start. We are trying to buckle up for the ride. We can't be in Joy's car, but we won't leave her alone on this ride. We don't know how many turns or how sharp they may be. We don't know how many climbs or how steep the falls will be. We all know that Joy's final roller coaster ride has probably started and will terminate sooner than later.

The uneventful weekend passed with Joy consuming almost no food or liquid. Her evenings were reportedly unsettled and unrestful. Every morning, we find her in a state between awake and asleep. Her mouth is open, her breath is shallow, and she is shifting between snores, gasps, and sudden body-shaking shutters. She paws at her gown and the IV connections on both wrists, clearly irritated by them. After some lengthy discussions with her medical team, we authorized her IV to be removed. They were a significant source of discomfort. She won't have an IV upon discharge. We needed to see if she would realize she needed to eat and drink without external support. The first main climb in this roller coaster ride has begun.

The body doesn't do well without food and, especially, liquid. A patient with Alzheimer's and dementia is stricken even harder. The body slows nutritional absorption and begins to burn residual body fat for energy. As dehydration advances, mental capacity declines, and in an already impaired mind, the patient forgets about eating or drinking. We followed Joy, where she took us.

As we crest the first twenty-four-hour mark without intravenous nutrition and hydration, Joy has had less than half a dozen bites of food and less than 250 ml of liquid. Knowing this, the medical team at the hospital spoke directly to Joy, with us by her side. They are recommending she return to her memory care apartment with hospice care. Joy listened quietly, said she wanted comfort care, and then started talking about sewing blankets together and selling them in New York. The medical team smiled. Joy smiled. Jan and I took a deep breath and swallowed hard. The roller coaster screamed down the tracks and hit a hard, poorly banked right turn at the bottom. The cars shoot through a spiral tube as Joy's mind becomes even more twisted and upside down. All the cars, one after another, begin to spin around, turning us upside down and righting us again, over and over.

We wrote Joy a message on her whiteboard: Joy, you fell and broke your hip. You are in the hospital and have had surgery. You are safe.

From her bed, Joy could read the note repeatedly. We hoped she could understand and that it would calm her. It did for a few days, and then we slipped through another spinning tube.

The message became, as Joy read it, "See, right there it says: 'Joy, you were pushed and broke your hip. You are in the hospital, and they aren't going to fix you. You are not safe. You've been had.'"

The message was erased as she slept; now, it shows only the date. After the next nap, she had forgotten the erased message altogether.

The rollercoaster exits the spiral, but Joy's mind and ours are spun around. The lift-hoist chain grabs the undercarriage of the cars, and whether we want to or not, we start up the next steep climb.

54
Hospice

The rollercoaster reaches another apex, slowing as the tow chain hauls our cars up and over. We free-fall along the tracks, wondering if they will hold as we careen down the other side into hospice care.

The transport from the hospital back to the memory care facility was uneventful, and Joy actually seemed to enjoy it. Strapped onto a gurney with a new, warm blanket covering her increasingly fragile body, she looked at us, smiled, and said she'd had a great vacation.

When she arrived, her room was ready for the new level of care. Her bed had been removed and replaced with an adjustable bed without rails. A fall mat folded up along the wall, a portable toilet, and a walker were also present. The hospice and memory care teams had pre-staged everything. Once Joy slid off the gurney and onto her "new" bed, she slipped into her dreamland, a place that now makes more sense than the reality swirling around her.

An onboarding hospice nurse talked us through the process while being interrupted every so often by Joy saying hello and dozing back off. The nurse confirmed what we already suspected. Unless there is a remarkable turnaround soon, Mom has little time left with us. That is hard to hear, even though Jan and I have said it to ourselves and one another several times in the past few days.

Joy is again disoriented. Her eldest son, my older brother, arrives. She blankly looks at us and then at him, then back at us. He greets her; she recognizes something in the sound of his voice and smiles. She has made a connection and is happy ... in that moment.

Her evening was spent running her fingers back and forth along the edge of her blanket over and over again. She kept saying, "I can't make it work. I have to cut it. I have to."

It was getting late in her day. We watched her frustration elevate. Her hands shook, her brow furrowed, and her eyes twitched. Each in our own way, we held her. Held her in our hearts. Joy would not relax, so we held her hand until the tension eased, and she dozed off.

The roller-coaster cars begin to slow as the end comes into sight. Time has no meaning. We wonder how slow the cars will go and how far they will travel before they come to a stop. Regardless, we will not leave her alone on the ride.

55
Waiting and Watching

As expecting parents, we waited with anxious anticipation for each of our son's birth, hoping they would be healthy. Now, we again wait in anxious anticipation for Joy's departure, hoping it will be painless. Each hospice nurse has confirmed that we are looking at days, not weeks before this roller-coaster ride rolls slowly to its end.

Mom seems to be comfortable as she lays in bed and tells mixed stories of reality and fantasy. A common theme is woven into Joy's monologue: she is happy, at peace, and thankful for her spouse and family. In a strong, yet pausing, voice she says:

"I'm squared away with my husband, my sons, their families, and myself. ... I'm home free. I'm not frightened anymore."

Jan and I listen. We laugh at some of her subsequent little jokes. All the while crying a little more inside. As we hold space for Mom and silently grieve for all she's endured and for our own loss, we're also keenly aware of the solemn reality before us.

We believe death isn't an end but rather a beginning we don't understand. It is a journey of the soul full of new adventures while a piece of her stays with us forever. Death is the great common denominator in life's equation. It is the one thing that cuts through and is shared by all of us, regardless of race, gender, orientation, politics, nationality, or status. Aside from birth, it is the one thing we all get to do.

For Joy, death will be a release from a broken mind and now a broken body. It will be a relief. After a rich, whole mortal life, Mom's soul is now at the precipice of a new, wondrous adventure. We sit by her bedside, silently waiting and watching. Letting her go will be hard for us, but keeping her would be cruel to her.

The human body is nothing short of miraculous. It knows when its time is ending and begins to shut down. Food and liquids are no longer being absorbed and can actually become harmful to the body, so appetite and thirst diminish. As the body efficiently uses its reserves, weight is steadily lost, and ketosis sets in. Dulled pain receptors induce a sense of euphoria, and calcium build-up leads to increased tiredness and more sleep. Joy's delusions and dementia seem heightened as her body slowly yields to the inevitable.

The clouds begin to fill the sky and bring a calming, filtered light into Joy's room. A light classical piano concert is playing, filling the room with tranquil tones. Joy's breathing is shallow, and she rests peacefully, body, mind, and soul. We wait and watch, not knowing whether this will be her last nap or a few more will follow. Either way, we find it impossible to leave. We silently reflect on Joy, her life, and her impact on us and our friends. Silently, each in our own way, we are trying to simultaneously hold her and let her go.

56
Vigil

We sit in an unknowing, anxious vigil. When we brought Joy from the hospital to her memory care apartment, the onboarding hospice nurse left us with the clear impression she was almost gone. Yet, seven days later, here we are, our vigil painfully extending one long day after another.

Joy continues her meager consumption trend. Over the last several days, she has had a few shrimps, some berries, and a few walnut halves, along with a few sips of liquid, usually with medication. We had originally hoped that returning to her apartment and its familiar faces and surroundings might spur her appetite, but it hasn't. She has lost ten to fifteen pounds during this ordeal.

Although Joy's dance with death is hard to watch, it is also inspiring. She drifts in and out of both worlds, never fully in either. Her dementia has increased, which isn't a surprise, given what she has survived. She sees things that aren't there and talks with loved ones who have gone before her. Out of nowhere, as she sleeps, she suddenly reaches her arms up as if greeting a long-lost friend or just needing to stretch, but we will never know which. She, again, fidgets with her sheet and blanket—folding, unfolding, measuring, and wrapping up her pillow in them.

Looking at us with an exasperated, silly grin, she'll say, "I just can't get these things to fold even. I just can't."

Then she tries again. At one point in this repetitive process, she silently decided she might have better results if her gown was also folded up with the sheets. We smile and help her keep a little bit of her dignity. Still, the darn sheet just won't fold straight.

After she visits with the hospice nurse and a caring bed bath, we resume our places by her bed. We have discovered that her field of vision is now severely limited. There seems to be no peripheral view, only direct. We take turns sitting in the "hot seat," always ready to give her a quick smile and our undivided attention.

Her pale, ashen face and gaping mouth are ghostly and haunting. At the same time, she seems at peace and serene. Her involuntary twitching, for the moment, is minimal. Her body is still, except for the shallow breaths, slightly raising her arms as they lay across her chest.

Sleep ... Sleep ... Sleep ...

It is complex and tiring to have a foot in each world. Yet, Joy has remained Joy throughout. She smiles and winks and is kind to the caregivers, as they are kind to her. She wants to please. She wants to help them help her.

Joy's journey, our journey, the journey many have followed, is ending. We don't know when, but we know it will. We think Joy knows, too. Joy has always been a guiding star for us and still is, even now. We sit quietly by her side and wait, as the classical piano music lofts through the air and Joy breathes calmly in her sleep. We are all at peace.

57
Slow Dance

Joy's waltz with the two worlds of life and death has become a slow dance, and no one really knows when the music will end. We sit by her bedside all day, as she drifts in and out of sleep. Sometimes, she looks peaceful, and other times, she is agitated, whether asleep or awake. But now she sleeps most of the day and night, with only brief intervals of being awake.

Her calm demeanor over the last week has changed. She has ever-increasing bouts of hallucinations. Most are pleasant; others are not. She sees ponies in the room or dancers around her bed. Then she sees a foot coming through the window or someone under the bed. She calls out for help, and when we take her hand, she mostly smiles and greets us.

At one point, she woke up with a start and called out, "What is happening to me? Just tell me. I'm so confused. I don't understand."

We held her hand as we explained that her body was trying to heal but was having an exceedingly challenging time. As we stroked her hair and gently rubbed her forehead, she looked up with confused, questioning eyes and shook her head.

"I'm so confused," she repeated. "I just don't understand."

Finally, she calmed down and dozed off again. We were left wondering whether we should tell her what was really happening. We opted not to.

Joy is now receiving some anti-anxiety medication to help during the agitated periods. So begins one more spin of the slow dance as the somber music plays.

Her breathing changes from deep, rapid, gasping draws of air to very shallow ones. Her mouth falls open most of the time now, as she appears unable to breathe through her nose. Her gasping can be alarming. It certainly gets our attention. We wait and watch, wondering if the gasp might be the last one or just another in a series of heart-wrenching, desperate breaths.

Joy's interest in food and drink continues to decline. Sometimes, we wonder if she eats or touches any of her meals. But then, unexpectedly, she will have a few bites and sips, just enough to stretch the slow dance out a few more stanzas. She apparently has lost all sense of taste, given that she chews her pain medication without flinching while the rest of us shudder to think of how vile the taste must be. All her food is now "finger food," as she can no longer manage a spoon or fork. Every caregiver is watching to see if swallowing is becoming difficult. When it becomes an incumbrance, her medication will be mixed into a syringe and gently released into the back of her mouth.

The genuinely kind, caring, and gentle hospice nurse suggested Joy has "about a week to go, unless she doesn't." The meager sustenance and her body's consumption of what reserves she still has can carry her forward a little longer. Her digestive organs and kidneys will soon begin to shut down, and she is no longer able to metabolize food or even water. The hospice doctor ordered the cessation of all eating and drinking by mouth. Metaphysically, we know this isn't sustainable. But the band keeps playing, and Joy keeps slowly dancing.

58
Advocacy

Joy's systolic blood pressure dropped thirty points over two days. She is hard to arouse with any stimulation and almost incoherent the little she speaks during the few moments she is awake. She continues to remain pleasant but much weaker. The hospice nurse told us Joy's body was telling us a lot. Joy's dance seemed to be winding down. ... And then it wasn't.

Without explanation, Joy has suddenly been much more alert and chattier, although still confused and confusing when speaking. The hospice nurse returned for her tri-weekly visit and reported Joy's blood pressure and other vitals had returned to normal. We must have had a blank look on our faces, but so did the nurse. Almost simultaneously, we noticed the urine collection bag and mentioned how much lighter and clearer her urine had appeared. We all took a deep sigh. We thought and the nurse confirmed there was only one way for that to occur: someone has been proactive in liquid support.

The hospice doctor's orders have been unambiguous. Joy is well past her life's tipping point. There is no expectation of recovery. Every little bite of food or encouraged liquid consumption is now harmful to Joy and not beneficial. In their zeal to give care, someone has misunderstood the orders or the impact of fudging on them. Joy's clock has been reset, and the only one hurt by this ingestion of food and encouraged liquid is Joy. It is difficult for her to swallow, and her digestive system can no longer process or tolerate food. Liquids slightly rehydrate her, only as a tantalizing tease to her system, allowing it to rebound slightly but without any sustainable duration.

We find ourselves across the Rubicon. There is no going back. After so many years and recently so many hard days of being her advocates for life, we are now Joy's advocates for the end of her life. It is a hard transition. A part of us had always hoped for some sort of recovery, but we are realistic and must be pragmatic. Our emotions can no longer sway our decisions other than to do whatever we can and must do to keep Joy comfortable.

Sadly, Joy remains a pleaser and will take whatever is offered to see a smile on someone's face. The hospice orders are clear: liquids only with medication unless Joy specifically requests it. The care staff struggles with these orders, and understandably so. They are trained to help and to give care. Several comment on how hard this is; "We love Joy and don't want her to go." We love her, too; therefore, we must let her go and ensure her comfort.

We post a sign on Joy's door for everyone who enters to read:

Joy has passed her life's tipping point. Love and care are now shown by helping us let her go with dignity.

This is hard. Every innocent action intended to help now harms. It is exceedingly difficult for people to shift and become end-of-life advocates when their hearts and training are focused on caring for life. Joy would never want to live the way she's had to in her final few days. She has endured indignities, pain, and situations she would never have wanted. Doing what we can to help her complete her life's journey as peacefully as possible is all we can do now.

Epilogue

Joy passed away, not from Alzheimer's, but because of two hip fractures and subsequent reparative surgeries. At ninety-one years old, the odds of surviving those events for almost two months, as she did, were less than 5 percent. Joy's Alzheimer's was a contributing factor in her inability to understand what was happening or where she was. She passed away with a broken body and a broken mind.

Although Joy's physical presence is gone, her spirit lives on. Her legacy and memories of her will last for many generations. We—her family, friends, caregivers, and all who knew Joy—are all the better for who she was and what she taught us about ourselves.

The last time Jan and I were with my mom, when she had any resemblance of cognitive ability, she opened her eyes as she lay in bed. She looked over, we smiled, and she smiled. Her eyes seemed clearer than usual, as she spoke weakly but clearly:

"Thank you. I love you."

She closed her eyes as we reached for her hand and told her we loved her too.

To all those who have joined us on our journey and for all those who will have their own journey:

Thank you. We love you. Have Courage, Be Bold, and **Never Fear the Dream**.

Memoriam

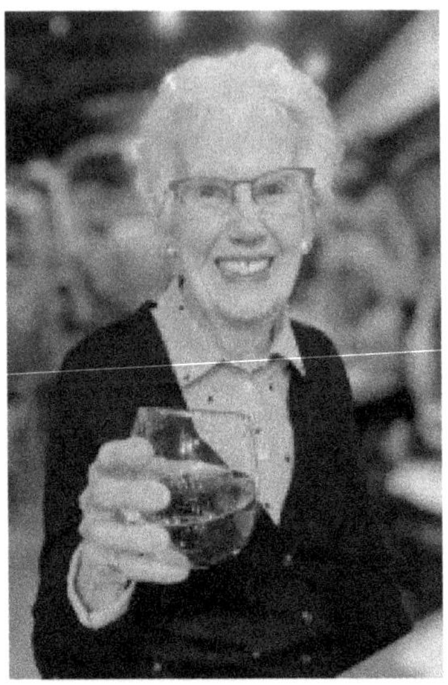

Joy was an amazing woman, friend, wife, and mother, grandmother, and great-grandmother. Her ninety-one years were filled with love for everyone she met, adventure, and a caring spirit right to the end. Joy passed on September 22, 2024. Among her final words were, "I'm the most blessed person in the world." We didn't have the heart to tell her it was us, all of us, whom she made the most blessed just by being herself and being part of our lives.

Joy was born in far West Texas in 1933, as the depression slowly ended. She grew up on a farm/ranch, learning to keep everything "just in case" and, more importantly, acceptance of others. Her playmates and friends on the ranch and at the small school she attended were of mixed races and religions. She imparted her conviction of acceptance to her sons, their friends, and hers.

Joy didn't just study the Bible; she lived its teachings. She brought her love of people, all people, to the Presbyterian Session and helped guide her church to be inclusive and welcoming, to teach lessons of life, and to be better neighbors. Joy often said she prayed twice because she was so engaged in the church choir.

Joy often said the only thing she ever wanted was to be a wife and mother. She was terrific at both. She was a dedicated, loving wife. She traveled the backroads of Texas, New Mexico, Arizona, and Wyoming, living and starting a family in a trailer with her life partner as he worked the mining fields and mineral exploration projects. These were her "nomad" years, which were sometimes lonely and hard but mostly filled with adventure and broadening experiences.

To us, she was the best mom and mom to our friends. To her grandchildren and great-grandchildren, she was the best Momo ever. She was always there. She always gave us a hand to hold when ours were scared and trembling. She always had kind, loving, supporting words for us, teaching us the lessons she felt she needed to impart. She took all our friends under her wing and gave them the same love and attention she gave us. She opened our home and welcomed anyone who needed a place to stay. She didn't care about gender, race, or religion; they were our friends, and therefore, they were her extra children, whom she loved.

Joy was an accomplished lady at a time when women weren't necessarily supposed to be. She earned a teaching degree and worked as a substitute teacher. Fifteen years after receiving her teaching degree, she returned to college, earning a Bachelor of Science in Library Science. Joy was a fantastic Cub Scout Den Mother and Eagle Scout Mentor. She was instrumental in converting the high school from a PTA to a PTSA, because she believed the students' opinions should be heard. Joy was a religious leader and one of the first women Deacons and Elders in the local Presbyterian church. She was an avid member of the Philanthropic Educational Organization (P.E.O.) for over 50 years. Joy strenuously advocated for a new neighborhood hospital and gave testimony before the Texas State Legislature. But Joy was most proud of being on the Board of Directors of the Lee Moor Children's Home in El Paso. She was a tireless advocate for the children and their future.

Joy also never turned down a glass of wine or a piece of Dove dark chocolate. Cheers, Joy!

Joy knew time with people was more special than any task. She spent time making a friend with everyone and helping whenever she could. Ironically, that helping hand became her downfall. She would be all right with that, if she were here and could remember. Joy lived with the idea that if you want to go fast, you go alone; if you want to go far, take someone with you. She took many of us by the hand and took us along on an incredible journey. A person's reach should be longer than their grasp. Joy's reach has touched so many and far beyond her grasp, and we are all so much better because of her. She will never be gone as long as we remember and tell her stories.

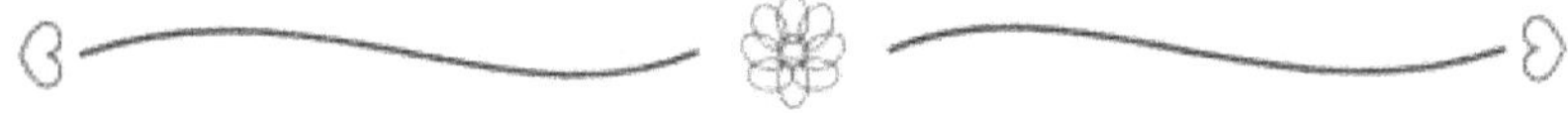

Afterword

Joy's story is familiar to our aging population. For those who suffer from Alzheimer's or any other form of dementia and mental affliction, their final years can be very difficult for both them and their loved ones. Every story is unique. Every story is personal. Every story should be told.

There is still a social stigma around mental illness and even mental health. While the stigma isn't as prevalent today as it once was, its heinous head continues to rise. We view someone in a wheelchair differently than someone with a mental health issue. It's easier for us to accept physical injury than mental illness. We're more comfortable with physical disabilities because we see them every day. Ironically, we encounter people with mental health issues daily and may not even realize it. But when we do recognize them, we often feel uncomfortable and frightened. It isn't anything they did to us; it's what we do to ourselves. Maybe, just maybe, we see a little of ourselves in them, remember a loved one, or cringe at the idea that we, too, might suffer a similar affliction. We don't understand mental illness, and so we shy away from and ignore what we can't fathom.

Mental health is rapidly becoming a significant issue for health and care facilities. Projections show the aging population, over 70 years, will make up as much as 20 percent of the US population by 2050. These facilities—whether assisted living, memory care, skilled nursing, or psychiatric—are unprepared for the current need and woefully unprepared for the coming tsunami. Mental health is critical. We need to address it head-on and not hide from it.

More importantly, we need to address the social and personal stigmas associated with mental illness and dementia from all causes. Until we begin to accept and respect those afflicted, we, as individuals and society, will never be able to care for, love, or cherish those who need our support the most. Modern medicine can fix most things that are broken in a body, but it cannot fix a broken mind. But there are ways to make the journey easier for people with mental illnesses and their loved ones. We can change our perception. We can be more caring, compassionate, and supportive. And we'd better change our ways because, odds are, all of us will experience some degree of cognitive decline as we age. We must learn these lessons ourselves and hope those around us will accept us as we are and who we will become. We must learn to advocate for continued-life care and end-of-life care with the same energy and passion.

Invitation

Jan and I invite everyone to join in the conversation and advocacy for all forms of mental health and dementia. These are real problems, and they will only worsen as our population grows and life's stress increase.

The following are some of the many organizations that can aid you in your efforts as a caregiver or as someone affected by Alzheimer's or other forms of dementia.

1. **Alzheimer's Association:** alz.org | 24/7 Helpline, 800–272–3900 | Provides education, support groups, resources, and a dynamic chat room.

1. **Alzheimer's Foundation of America (AFA):** alzfdn.org | National Toll-Free Helpline 866–232–8484

1. **Dementia Society of America:** dementiasociety.org | Toll-free: 1–800–DEMENTIA

1. Mental Health America (MHA): mhanational.org

1. National Alliance on Mental Illness (NAMI): nami.org | Help Line, 800–950–6264

1. National Institute of Mental Health (NIMH): nimh.nih.gov

Numerous books and literature on the subject exist, several of which resonated with us on our journey and are cited earlier in this book. We encourage you to read and research as much and as often as you can. While many of the books are for professional caregivers, some, like Joy in Alzheimer's, address the journey from the perspective of a loved one or, more rarely, the person with dementia.

While Alzheimer's and other forms of dementia may not be curable today, this should not discourage us from becoming engaged and supportive. We can make a difference, even if it is one person at a time.

By knowing more, we can make that one person's life a little easier. It will also make your life easier in a demanding situation.

Please join in the effort and make a difference.

My blog, simplebender.com, is always open for comments, dialogue, and article suggestions.

Have Courage, Be Bold, and Never Fear the Dream

About the Author

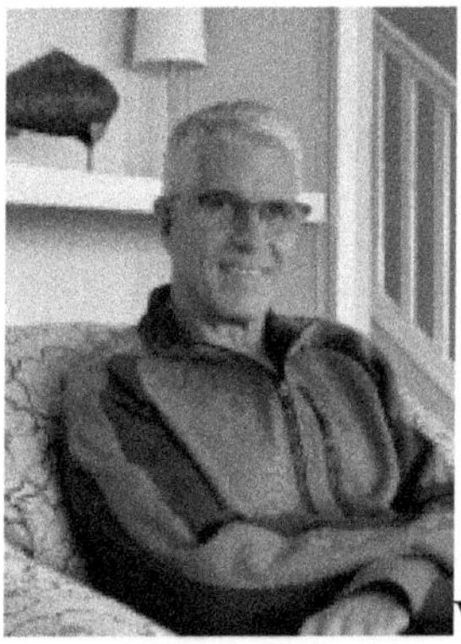

William C. Barron and his wife, Jan, followed and aided his mother, Joy, on her Alzheimer's journey, documenting it as they went along. William authored the book's episodes in real-time while incorporating clinical and caregiver resources to aid others on their journey.

The author has written and published several technical articles and is a frequent guest columnist in local news media. His blog, **simplebender.com**, has attracted audiences across the United States, Canada, Europe, and Asia.

William is a retired petroleum engineer who has worked professionally on three continents, above the Arctic, and below the Equator. He worked as an offshore roustabout, engineer, and operations manager. He was a senior corporate executive before becoming the State of Alaska's Oil and Gas Division Director. He is currently the Principal at Trispectrum Consulting. He co-holds many patents and has many years of public speaking experience and State Legislative testimony.

William is an accomplished endurance athlete who has been on Team USA for several World Championship ITU Duathlons, completed numerous half-Ironman and Ironman events, and completed the Boston Marathon.

Did you love *Joy in Alzheimer's*? Then you should read *Lap Around the Sun*[1] by William Barron!

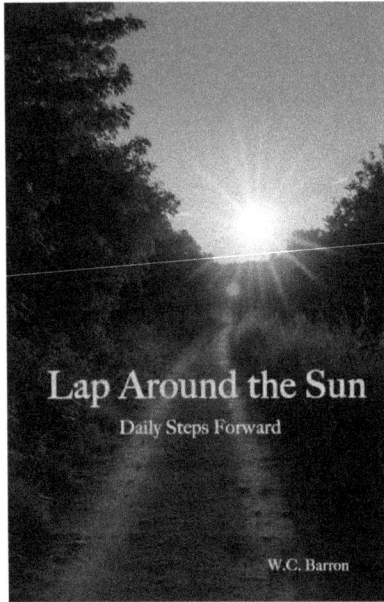

[2]

Discover a unifying journey through humanity's greatest wisdom traditions with Lap Around the Sun: Daily Steps Forward. This daily companion transcends cultural and philosophical boundaries, weaving together the profound insights of Eastern contemplation, Western rational thought, and African communal wisdom into a harmonious collage of human understanding.

- Benefit: Find a deeper understanding of yourself and your place in the world

- Change Your Life: Embrace your circumstances, face life's challenges with wisdom and grace, and find purpose and connection in every moment.

---

1. https://books2read.com/u/3JAP5P
2. https://books2read.com/u/3JAP5P

- The book is organized around eight core themes, including Amor Fati, Mortality, Emotion, and Resilience, providing a comprehensive framework for personal growth.

- Each daily contemplation begins with a powerful quote or principle, followed by a thoughtful narrative that unpacks its meaning for contemporary life.

- The book integrates diverse philosophical traditions, revealing their underlying connections and universal truths.

- Practical tools for navigating life's challenges and opportunities are provided in the Action, Problem Solving, and Resilience sections.

- The book serves as a compass for your life's journey and a unique tool for personal transformation and spiritual growth.

Embark on a journey of self-discovery and personal growth. Lap Around the Sun is more than just an inspirational, motivational book, it is a compass for your life's journey and a unique tool for personal transformation and spiritual growth. This book is for you whether you're a young professional seeking meaning in your career, a middle-aged adult navigating life transitions, or someone hungry for a deeper understanding of yourself and your place in the world.

In this book, you'll find:

- Guidance on embracing your circumstances and finding purpose in every moment.

- Wisdom and insights that will touch your soul and inspire personal growth.

- A comprehensive framework for personal growth, organized around eight core themes.

- Practical tools for navigating life's challenges and opportunities.

- Daily contemplations that can be read in any order, offering fresh insights and inspiration with each reading.

- A journey through the different seasons of life, helping you find purpose and connection in every precious, unrepeatable moment.

Don't wait any longer to start your journey towards personal growth and spiritual transformation.

Read more at simplebender.com.

Also by William Barron

Joy in Alzheimer's
Lap Around the Sun

Watch for more at simplebender.com.

www.ingramcontent.com/pod-product-compliance
Lightning Source LLC
Chambersburg PA
CBHW031219290326
41931CB00035B/421
* 9 7 9 8 9 9 8 7 6 9 5 1 1 *